T0098501

||||||||||||||||||||||||||||||||||||||||||||||

Advance Praise

"Debbie Lazinsky's *No Time to Lose* is a wonderful blend of practical wisdom, real world tools, and inspiration on how to change your perspective on weight loss. Her personal story leaves no doubt that she has run the race and figured out how to win – no matter how many times you may have dropped out in the past."

–Thomas M. Sterner author of *The Practicing Mind*

"The power of Debbie Lazinsky's book, *No Time to Lose*, lies in its honesty, simplicity, and no-nonsense approach. Not just another "how to lose weight" book, and definitely not another fad diet, *No Time To Lose* is a testament to the human mind and spirit. Make sure you pay close attention to the lemon lesson."

–Karen C.L. Anderson, Master Certified Life Coach and author of *The Peaceful Daughter's Guide To Separating From A Difficult Mother*

NO TIME TO LOSE

NO TIME
TO LOSE

Debbie LAZINSKY

NEW YORK

NASHVILLE • MELBOURNE • VANCOUVER

No Time to Lose

How I Lost 185 Pounds and Saved My Life

© 2018 Debbie Lazinsky

All rights reserved. No portion of this book may be reproduced, stored in a retrieval system, or transmitted in any form or by any means—electronic, mechanical, photocopy, recording, scanning, or other—except for brief quotations in critical reviews or articles, without the prior written permission of the publisher.

Published in New York, New York, by Morgan James Publishing in partnership with Difference Press. Morgan James is a trademark of Morgan James, LLC. www.MorganJamesPublishing.com

The Morgan James Speakers Group can bring authors to your live event. For more information or to book an event visit The Morgan James Speakers Group at www.TheMorganJamesSpeakersGroup.com.

ISBN 9781683504047 paperback
ISBN 9781683504054 eBook
Library of Congress Control Number: 2017900725

Cover and Interior Design by:
Chris Treccani
www.3dogdesign.net

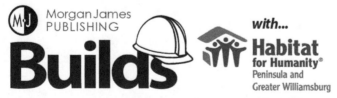

In an effort to support local communities, raise awareness and funds, Morgan James Publishing donates a percentage of all book sales for the life of each book to Habitat for Humanity Peninsula and Greater Williamsburg.

Get involved today! Visit
www.MorganJamesBuilds.com

‖‖‖‖‖‖‖‖‖‖‖‖‖‖‖‖‖‖‖‖‖‖‖‖‖‖‖

Disclaimer

Neither the author nor the publisher assumes any responsibility for errors, omissions, or contrary interpretations of the subject matter herein. Any perceived slight of any individual or organization is purely unintentional.

Brand and product names are trademarks or registered trademarks of their respective owners.

The names and other identifying characteristics of the persons included in this book have been changed. Throughout this book the author has used examples from many clients' lives. However, to ensure privacy and confidentiality their names and some of the details of their experiences have been changed. All of the personal examples of the author's own life have not been altered.

This book contains discussions about health issues and weight loss. While the author may have her own opinions about these topics, they are just that- opinions based on training, skills and personal experience. The author is not a physician and advises you to ask your physician if you have any questions about your health. In addition, please note that the author cannot be held responsible for medical decisions that you make as a result of reading this book. Please contact your physician before undertaking any of the recommendations made here.

||||||||||||||||||||||||

Dedication

To Neil,
for loving me through thick and thin.

||||||||||||||||||||||||||||||||||||||||||||

Table of Contents

||||||||||||||||||||||||||||||||||

Introduction

I set out to lose weight to save my life. I never expected to be included in *People* magazine's "Half Their Size" issue. It was such a thrill to be selected for that honor. Being super sensitive about having my picture taken was a big obstacle that I had to overcome before I could even imagine doing it.

I was astounded when I was contacted by the editors at *People*. I really thought it was a friend playing a joke on me. But it was real, and soon I was sending *before* and *after* photos to the editors and doing phone interviews. Then they told me they'd get back to me, so I figured that was the end of it. Much to my surprise, the call came in around Thanksgiving that I should be prepared to get to California in the first week of December (this was in 2013), because I was one of the five winners who would be featured in their biggest story in the "Half Their Size" issue, and I was going to be a centerfold model (OMG!?). *And* they were picking up the expense. Wow!

Off I went, not knowing what to expect. I had spent my career in advertising and marketing, so I was no stranger to a professional TV and photo shoot. Except this time I was in front of the camera and not giving direction from behind it. But there I was with my four new friends who were also in that issue: Kodi, Kate, Ginger, and Sheree. We all came from different parts of the country; we were of varying ages and ethnicities; and, on the surface, we could not have been a more diverse group. Yet, underneath, we shared the same battle and victory over our weight. I was the oldest, by far – close to twice the age of the others.

The entire experience was magical.

We did the photoshoot at the former estate of celebrity Dinah Shore. We had a truly world-class photographer in Troy Word, who made us look (even more) beautiful. Google him and check out his work. The entire *People* team was absolutely wonderful.

We were sworn to secrecy and couldn't post any of the photos that had been shot that weekend in early December, so by the time the issue was released in early January, I was about to burst with anticipation. The magazine came out and it was on every newsstand in New York and everywhere else *People* is sold. It was crazy. We were on national TV shows, like *Extra* and *Inside Edition*, and also on local and national TV news. The issue was featured all over the world.

It's been a few years since the magazine came out. I still get a thrill when I think of that weekend when the issue came out and the recognition it brought to my message. I realized that the reason I was able to overcome my fear of having my picture taken wasn't because I was in the care of an über professional hair stylist, makeup artist, and photographer; it was because I felt a responsibility to share my story with women all over the world. That was much more powerful to me than my fear of having my picture taken.

The number one question I get when women see the magazine and contact me or find out I was in it is "How did you do it?!"

This book is the answer.

‖‖‖‖‖‖‖‖‖‖‖‖‖‖‖‖‖‖‖‖‖‖‖‖

Chapter 1
Here's the Truth

My goal is to teach you the tools you need to successfully manage your weight for your lifetime. You can live the life you deserve once you understand a few facts and are willing to face the truth.

So let me give it to you straight. The reason you are overweight is because your calorie burn is less than your calorie consumption. Yup! It's all about the bottom line. When your calorie net is zero, your weight stays the same. A surplus in cash is great, but in calories, not so much. We're looking for a deficit in order to move the number on the scale downward.

This is where I lose a lot of people, so if you're still with me, congratulations! You have faced the first truth.

As you read this book, I will give you some tools and ideas to help make getting to the deficit easier than ever before.

How Much Do You Want This?

I've taken hundreds and hundreds of women through this process. Those who are willing to put in the effort are successful, and not only in getting the body they desire. They now take far fewer medicines and have boundless energy. They also take their new found confidence and use it in every aspect of their lives to do things like asking for a promotion, taking on a big assignment, making a big change in their relationship, or going back to school. They start to live the life they're supposed to be living, following their dreams and accomplishing great stuff. But you have to want this enough to stick with the process. Be honest with yourself and answer this question: Are you truly ready to do what it takes to accomplish your goal?

Meet Mary

Mary is a 48-year-old single woman who is an avid exerciser. She has a great job and a bubbly personality. She's 100 pounds overweight and believes she is cursed to never be able to lose the excess weight. On the other hand, she desperately wants a man in her life, but feels like no man will want her until she loses the weight. She passes up dates with guys who ask her out because she questions their motives. *Why would he want to date me except for easy sex?* So she doesn't date at all.

Life is passing her by while she's waiting for the right number to show up on the scale. She won't be seen in a bathing suit, so she doesn't go to the beach anymore, even though she loves the beach, and times spent at the beach make up some of her happiest childhood memories. She won't visit her relatives in Germany because those airplane seat belts are so small and asking for a seat belt extender is out of the question. And forget about being in her friends' wedding parties. *Ugh*. That is too much hurt in one place. She'd have to buy a dress and stand next to four other skinny girls and be the fattest one in the pictures, the one who will probably never get married.

There's a constant dialog running in Mary's head. She's always coming up with excuses so she doesn't have to face the truth. It's exhausting, and it's easier to stay home.

Life is passing her by.

The day Mary decided to be completely honest with herself was the day she started her final weight loss journey.

What Works for You?

Succeeding at permanent weight loss is about far more than the number of calories you eat or crunches you do. It is quite rare to lose more than 30 pounds and keep it off, with 98% of those who lose weight regaining what they've lost – and more. Like many women, I've lost the same pounds over and over again. In fact, at one point, I had lost 125 pounds by eating only the tiniest amount of calories and exercising like crazy. I regained it all, plus another 60 pounds, and I don't remember at all doing that. I carried those extra 185 pounds for another 15 years.

I want you to know that each of us has a unique formula for successful weight management, and you can find yours when you know where to look for the answers.

We Are What We Think

If knowledge about how much food to eat and exercise was all we needed to control our weight, it would be great. Even when we understand this equation and the reasons for maintaining a healthy weight, we still find it difficult or almost impossible to accomplish. It doesn't matter how smart you are or where you are in your company's organizational chart. Fat is an equal opportunity employer. You can't just decide to eat less and move more and think the problem is solved. You've got lots of old habits and beliefs that will pull you back into your old ways if you try to do this by willpower alone.

Weight management, as I tell my clients (with apologies to Yogi Berra), is 50% about what you eat and 80% about how you think, but it does not have to be a struggle or a battle. It does not mean that you have to starve, give up all your favorite foods, lose your identity, or wait to start living until you've lost the weight. In fact – and you may find this difficult to believe – you can eat more and still reduce your total caloric intake (this is a concept I will teach you about later).

Don't Be Fooled

Billions of dollars are invested by the marketers of diet programs and diet remedies to convince you that you can only be successful if you buy their shakes or go to their meetings. Now that bariatric surgery has become mainstream, some people would have you believe that it is the final answer. But it's not.

A large group of my clients have had bariatric surgery and are working with me because their weight has started to creep back. They thought the surgery was their last resort, the final solution to their weight problem. I can't imagine putting all of my hopes into having bariatric surgery only to find my weight climbing again. I especially want to give you hope if this sounds familiar to you.

You Can Find Your Way Out

As an intelligent, successful business woman, you juggle a whole bunch of stuff every day and leave your needs for last. I know how it feels to be so depleted at the end of the day that food has become a major source of joy, relaxation, and escape. You wish to wake up thin tomorrow, but the pain of knowing it's not going to happen can drive you to Ben & Jerry's for consolation. You're like that hamster on the wheel, always running and getting nowhere. How could the very thing that brings you so much relief and enjoyment be causing you so much pain? *Why can't I just be normal and eat like everyone else? There must be something genetically wrong with me.* Those were my thoughts, and I also hear those thoughts daily from my clients of every shape, age, and size. It doesn't matter if they want to lose ten pounds or 200 pounds – their thoughts are startlingly similar.

When you're stuck on that hamster wheel, it seems impossible to think you can ever really be successful. I was caught in that spin cycle a few years ago. I was a successful executive who always had a smile on my face and a solution for everyone who had a problem. But behind that smile was someone who longed to travel the world, eat great food on a daily basis, and shop for clothing anywhere but Lane Bryant.

I learned how to escape that spin cycle. It wasn't easy. I had to first learn what to feed my body, then I had to learn why I made the food choices I had been making. Ultimately I learned that food took up too much of my life and my thinking. It became obvious to me that in order to save my life, I needed to develop a new relationship with food.

I will take you through the five elements necessary to reach and maintain your ideal weight and start living your future life today. This process will change your relationship with food forever. There is no time to waste and there's no point in waiting.

|||||||||||||||||||||||||||||

Chapter 2
I Lost 185 Pounds
on My Own

'm sure I was born with a spoon in one hand and a book in the other. To say that I've had a lifelong struggle with weight sounds so cliché but, in my case, my weight was what defined me and every decision I made, from the time of my earliest memories. My relationship with food was intertwined with love, family, and acceptance. Food was my currency, my friend, my entertainment. All of my fondest memories and the biggest events in my life were celebrated with or centered on food. I love to cook and I love great food.

Through my childhood, well-meaning adults would try to bribe, beg, or manipulate me into eating less. There were threats, ultimatums, meltdowns, and, finally, no communications at all.

It Started in the First Grade

I can remember being in the first grade and being taken out of class once a week for a special club that the school nurse had created for a few kids like me who were chubbier than the rest. At first it made me feel special, but then we were forced to get on the scale and the nurse would either congratulate us and give us a safety pin for each pound we lost, or she'd sternly warn us that we weren't doing things right. In her view, it was a badge of honor to put on those safety pins each morning and wear them at school every day. I found it humiliating and refused to wear those stupid safety pins.

Of course my parents weren't happy about my weight. They took me to a doctor who prescribed "diet pills" (that was in 1962) and told me, "If you don't take them and lose weight, one day you'll be a 300-pounder." Those were his words. I can still see him and the office Mom and I were in when his opinion landed on me like a ton of bricks. And even though I assumed he was right, I hated the way those pills made me feel all jittery, and I hated the fact that nothing else I did made my parents happy if I wasn't dieting.

If Only I Could Be Perfect

I tried everything I could to be the perfect daughter, thinking maybe if everything else was *just right*, my parents would let me slide on my weight. I was a straight-A student for most of my school years. I can remember bringing home a report card that had all A's, but showed that I was absent three times, so that wasn't good enough. My takeaway as a child was that unless I was a certain weight on the scale or a certain dress size, then I was not lovable; I was not good enough.

That pattern repeated itself over and over again. I was the model employee, running circles around everyone else and quickly climbing the corporate ladder, always trying to prove I was good enough –

well, except for my weight, of course. As long as I did a great job, maybe no one would notice that I had become that 300-pounder the doctor had predicted.

I thought being a perfectionist was the answer. But I felt like an impostor. How could I be so good at school, at my job, and at just about anything I focused on – except my own body? Maybe I was a freak, genetically unable to lose weight, or was broken in some unfixable way. After all, the doctor had told me when I was seven how much I would weigh and there I was at 54 years old, standing on the scale staring at *318* in flashing red neon. *OMG! How will I lose 200 pounds?* was my first thought.

I went to the doctor, who told me, "If you don't have bariatric surgery, you won't live to see your 60th birthday."

Sentenced to Die

Holy smokes! I've got less than six years to live.

I went for the bariatric surgery consultation and knew it wasn't for me, but I also knew that although I had ignored this type of advice for 47 years, it was time to do *something*, but I had no idea where to start.

I waited another year before I actually took action, and I can remember the pivotal moment when I made the decision to live. It wasn't about fitting into a dress for a wedding or losing weight to meet a guy; it was about how many Christmases I had left, how many places I wanted to visit, and all the things I wanted to do but couldn't, because my weight was an obstacle. I had spent my entire life waiting to lose weight so that I could start living. Now my life was about to end and I still had so much I wanted to experience. My lowest moment came when I realized that I may as well be lying in ICU on life support, because all I was capable of doing was eating and breathing. I felt I had no right to breathe the air or take up space on the planet. I won't say I was suicidal, but I surely saw no reason to live at that point. My life was for nothing. I would die and no one would even know I had lived.

The Debbie Project

Even at my very lowest point, somehow, I remembered that I always came through on big projects at work, I successfully managed a 52-million-dollar advertising budget, and was great at my job. I was a super student. I had been offered full academic scholarships to some big, important universities. I wasn't stupid or lazy. So what was I missing?

I decided to treat myself as a work project. I imagined my boss coming to me and challenging me to do the impossible (as he loved to do, just to see what rabbit I could pull out of my hat). Since my goal was to prove that I could do anything, despite my weight, at work I would always rise to the occasion and over-deliver – under budget and ahead of schedule. I was always seeking perfection, praise, and acceptance, and hoping no one would call me out on my weight.

And so it began. I turned my weight loss into a work assignment and applied the corporate skills and experience I had mastered over 25 years and combined it with what I knew was not going to ever change about me, to see if I could fix myself once and for all.

This Time Will Be Different

It was going to be different this time. This time I was going to use my brain instead of trying to use will power or someone else's idea of what and how I should eat. Using my brain was the best decision I could have made, and the only method I had never tried. It had never occurred to me that I could *think* my way out of the early grave I had dug for myself.

I made a commitment to be honest with myself and to not accept any more BS excuses for why I couldn't get this job done.

I took a good look at where I was and where I hoped to finish. "Ironically," I told people, "I just want to live a healthier life. I'm not looking to be a bikini model or a centerfold." So how crazy is it that after 18 months of focused effort, I had lost those 185 pounds and was featured in the January 2014 issue of *People* magazine's "Half My Size" issue. And, yes, I was in the centerfold, with my clothes on!

I lost the weight and I've kept it off but, more importantly, along the way, I found myself, I learned that I am good enough, and I forgave my father for his misguided attempts to help me (although he died in 1977). Most importantly, I forgave myself.

A Funny Story about My Dad

My father didn't live to see me living my life at a healthy weight, but on the way to the *People* magazine shoot (which took place at Dinah Shore's former Palm Springs home), I stopped to stay with my mom at her new house in Phoenix.

Mom insisted that I sleep in her bed and she would sleep in the guest room. When it was time for bed, Mom asked me to sleep on the opposite side of the bed she usually slept on and told me to fold the bedspread over to the other side before I got into bed. I didn't know why she asked me to do that, and it didn't matter why, so I did what I she asked without question. I carefully folded the bedspread to the other side, got in bed and fell asleep.

I woke during the night and found that the bedspread had been unfolded and was covering me. I felt the warmth of a hug run through my body thinking what a "mommy thing" that was to do for your 59-year-old daughter, tucking her in. It was a nice warm feeling that I can still feel when I recall that moment.

Well, in the morning, over coffee, I thanked mom for covering me up and tucking me in. She said that when she checked on me before she went to bed I was sleeping with the bedspread folded over just like she had asked and she never got up to cover me or tuck me in.

I've decided to believe that was my dad, finally acknowledging that he is proud of me. That was a huge moment for me.

My Calling

At about 60 pounds down toward my goal, I started to feel guilty that the process was no longer taking up too much of my thoughts or time. I thought I had lost "it" – whatever it was that was allowing me to lose weight – and was afraid to weigh myself at the end of that month. I did anyway, and when I saw that I had lost ten pounds, just like I'd lost in each of the five months before, I realized that it was getting easy because I had developed new habits.

Habits are actions we do without much thought. Wow! Major discovery. I could train my brain to help me lose weight,. Who knew? I decided I had to tell everyone about it. I became determined to let the world know that successful weight loss doesn't have to be a daily struggle. New, healthy habits can begin to crowd out the old ones.

As long as you keep your goals in sight and use them to guide your choices, *the process will get easier*. That's what you've got to love about your habits: they take over.

But who would believe me if I talked about that with still another 130 pounds to lose? So I kept plugging away, relying on my plan, working and refining it along the way, always knowing I would not stop until I delivered on my Debbie Project goal.

Chapter 3

There Is Hope

I know how hard you've worked to lose weight in the past and what a sore subject this is to you, so I want to give you hope. I want you to know that there is a way to end this battle once and for all – and it's not a diet, I promise. We all know that diets don't work, and you don't need to be treated like a child who needs a time-out for eating too much.

Thank goodness you've ruled out any medical issues considering how long you've been yo-yo dieting. Although, secretly, you were hoping the doctor discovered you have a rare genetic disorder or some weird illness causing you to gain weight as you walk past a bakery or watch The Food Channel.

Heaven knows you've tried all the newest diets and programs and, year after year, your weight just keeps climbing. No, your clothes aren't shrinking by hanging in your closet. You're a wounded veteran of the diet wars, caught in the crossfire between Jenny, Weight Watchers, Paleo, and gluten-free. I know you're worn out and skeptical of the empty promises and the cost of awful tasting foods that leave you feeling empty. It's just too hard to stick with these programs for very long and, no matter what, the weight comes back as soon as you stop buying that stuff.

Let's Try Something New

Because I wish for you to shine as the intelligent, caring, and capable woman that you are, I'd like to invite you to take a fresh approach. Nothing else has worked in the past, so why not? Especially since my suggestion requires no big investment of time or money. It almost sounds too good to be true, doesn't it? And that is what's so ironic, because what I'm proposing is so simple that your first reaction is "This can't possibly work." But hear me out. Let me give you what worked for me. I lost 185 pounds and have kept it off doing exactly what I will describe to you, step by step, in this book.

Question Everything

Let's start with a clean slate and figure out what you need for your body to be happy and healthy, and then build the lifestyle to support that. This means I want you to be willing to question all of the diet advice you are bombarded with daily and question it. *Is this really true, what they offer? Or is this just another clever marketing tool to give me false hope and certain failure?* There is no shortage of bad diet information out there and those myths that they perpetuate need to go.

In fact, I wish you would question everything you believe about what and how you should eat. Where did those beliefs come from?

Are your stories accurate? After all, your beliefs, whether they are true or not, form the foundation for your identity.

You deserve the truth. You are entitled to this information.

Once we have the facts, we can create a strategy.

The Linda Project

Imagine that your name is Linda and your boss just handed you a file labeled "The Linda Project." Your assignment is to create a healthy, realistic, maintainable lifestyle for her. How would you approach that project? Where would you start?

Can you see how framing this as a work project given to you by someone who has faith in your abilities changes your thinking? How that one question – *Where would you start?* – opens your mind to possibilities? This is a very powerful lesson. Simply asking yourself the same questions in a new way changes your thinking immediately.

You'd likely approach this project by first assessing and gathering facts – not fretting over how impossible a task it will be to accomplish, or that it can't be done. You *know* this project will get done. It is inevitable. You may not yet know how or when it will get done, but there is no question in your mind that you will find a way to deliver. That's your job. That's why you get a paycheck. And so it's merely a question of *when* not *how*. No drama, just a bunch of to-do's. That's *why* this project will get done.

Use Your Executive Mind

Apply the same executive mindset that you've used to successfully propel yourself up the corporate ladder; the same skills you use daily to break down big, complex business projects into small, measurable, attainable, and realistic goals.

You already have these skills, my dear. You are so good at using them in your job and in your family life. I want to help you refocus those skills on the most important project of your life – *you*. You need to create that same sense of priority for *this* project and you will be successful. It's inevitable.

Find a Compelling Reason Why

Why do *you* want to lose weight? This may seem like a silly question. Yes, we all can recite the Surgeon General's warning about cigarettes, and yet millions of people still smoke. They *want* to quit, but they try unsuccessfully over and over again. Similarly, we all know that being overweight leads to all sorts of terrible illnesses that can eventually kill us just like cigarettes can. And yet the majority of our population in America is overweight.

Everyone I meet usually gets around to asking me what made me decide to lose weight and really do it? Wasn't it easier to just be fat?

Neither my father nor my grandfather made it to 50 years old, but that wasn't convincing enough for me. When my doctor told me I had six years left if I didn't lose weight, I still waited another year before I made up my mind to do something about it.

Knowing this stuff is meaningless until you find *your* compelling reason why getting your health in order needs to top your priority list. Once I did that, taking action on it became my number one focus in life.

Ask yourself this question and be totally honest when you answer: Do you really want to go through the process of steady, permanent weight loss, or do you want to be thin? This is an important question that deserves a thoughtful answer. Is your reason compelling enough to motivate you to see this project through? You're not getting a paycheck from someone else, so what will you get for your efforts? It's got to be *big* or this won't work.

Find your compelling reason why this project (you) deserves the time and attention it will take to learn some new skills and habits.

Start with the End in Sight

Let's get that executive brain of yours working on visualizing the final outcome of this project. Every project has to have a goal, right? So what is your vision? Can you see yourself living in a healthier body? Imagine being able to shop for new clothes in any clothing store instead of only a few stores or online? How about walking into a meeting confident about how you look and feel, so that the work you came to present isn't diminished by you worrying about your appearance? How would it feel to not give any thought to who may be judging you? How cool would that be? Imagine how it would feel to be free of the internal dialogue of doubt.

You can do this. I know you can. You've already proved to yourself and the world that you can do hard things. But you know that, in order to be successful at pulling off a big project at work, it takes time, planning, information-gathering, a support team, goal-setting, flexibility, accountability, and tenacity. You know this stuff.

Be Nice

My first request is for you to stop beating yourself up over your past diet history. The attempts you made were sincere, but they were also doomed to fail. *It's not your fault.* You have not been dealing with the real facts you needed to make the best choices. Your past attempts never got to the root of why you have the eating habits you do or why food occupies such a major role in your enjoyment of life.

You've been fighting against your body instead of working together with it as a team. How much could you get from your staff if all you ever did was bark at them about what stupid failures they were? Would they be productive and effective at their work? Could you count on them when times got tough to pull you through to meet a deadline or to think on their feet to recover from a crisis? No way. They'd be out of there in a heartbeat.

So, please, stop, take a breath, and commit to being kind to yourself. Promise?

To Do

Do a count of the frequency of the negative thoughts you have in a day. Anytime you look in the mirror or are unhappy with the scale, capture that thought and notice how you *feel* when you think it. I want you to become aware of how often you say negative things to yourself, things you'd never say to a friend or co-worker, yet you tolerate from yourself. This is not helpful to you in any way. At the end of the day, look at your count. You'll be astounded at how often you do this to yourself. Ask yourself how this serves you or if, perhaps, this daily beating is taking you further from your goals.

IIIIIIIIIIIIIIIIIIIIIIIIIIII

Chapter 4

A Fresh Approach

I created a fresh, new program to teach my clients how to simply achieve the life balance they seek. There are five elements I want to teach you about: food, rest, exercise, stress-management, and hydration.

As I do the program for myself, I like to think of managing these elements as keeping my ducks in a row, all swimming along in harmony. Every day, one or the other of them will get out of line if I stop paying attention. It's my job to watch out for this and apply my skills to which ever duck is acting out, so I can get it back in line and we can move along. In this way, I balance my life to reach my greatest potential.

My clients like to blame their eating habits for how much they weigh and how tired they feel, but they often don't realize that the headache they have may be due to dehydration, or their appetite can be affected by lack of sleep, or their mindset can create joy as well as misery. We are an entire organism, with many complex systems constantly at work supporting each other. None of the five elements can be separated from the rest if you want to have balance in your life. If you pay too much attention to one, the others will fall out of line. It's as if we have only a limited supply of focus to spread around and we need to keep a constant eye on the attention each element receives.

Five Key Elements

In the next chapters, we'll explore the role and importance of each FRESH element to see what a balanced life looks like. How much of each element do you have in line now? What would be ideal? We'll look at how to achieve a balance that works for you and how to create new habits, keep track, stay the course, test and measure, and refine.

The FRESH elements:

- *F*ood
- *R*est
- *E*xercise
- *S*tress Management
- *H*ydration

Where Are You Now and How Did You Get Here?

If you find yourself unhappy with the number on the scale or how your clothes fit, I want to make sure you understand that you didn't get here overnight. The reason you are *everything that you are* at this moment in time has much to do with the choices you've made over and over again. Many of those choices didn't even seem like choices if you've done them all your life.

Think about the family traditions about food that you grew up with. Wasn't it funny when you went out into the world and realized that not every family ate the same way yours did? We had dinner at 5:30 every night with a loaf of Italian bread on the table. How about when you encountered the cultural differences of people who ate foods for breakfast that made you squirm at the mere thought? *Fish for breakfast? No way, not me.* In our house when I was growing up, Sunday breakfast was pancakes, waffles, or French toast, and we had cereal on school mornings. That's what I did as an adult; until I met my husband and he introduced me to lox on a bagel! Who knew?

Suffice it to say that there are lots of big and small habits that you have cultivated over a lifetime about your food that should be examined and evaluated. We are on a mission to learn the truth as part of your research for your project, to find the habits that are working – so you can keep them – and to uncover those that are taking you further from your goals – so you can revise them. It's time to question everything. Don't stop asking *why* until you get a satisfactory answer. Remember that this is important business and we won't settle for an answer of "I don't know".

Since we are in information-gathering mode, ask yourself if you are eating when you're bored, tired, angry, happy, or sad. If the answer is *yes*, don't be surprised that you are in the majority. If you can truly answer *no*, your feelings never effect how much or how often you eat, or your choices of foods, then you are in the very small minority of people who simply need the facts about what and how they are eating and to create their formula for success. For those few, this process is simply a mathematical equation that I can teach in one hour. If this is you, then you will have the power to manage your weight for the rest of your life. Seriously.

Don't Be Afraid to Try New Things

Think about why you want to lose weight. What will be different? Are you willing to put in the effort? What will be better? Might some things be worse?

Changing the shape of your body forever is a really big deal. Trust me! Life is very different since I stopped carrying around that extra 185 pounds. It's like no longer going through life carrying a brother on your back. It was exhausting.

And now it's not.

Baby Steps

I'll never forget that snowy morning on January 2, 2009. That was the day I fully committed myself to losing the weight, once and forever. I was going to do it.

I dragged myself to the brand new gym in town that was opening that day. The snow was really coming down, but I arrived at the gym all fired up and ready to go. The place was dark and the door was locked, but I could see a guy in the back turning the lights on. He waved me away and told me the gym wasn't opening for another half-hour. But then I guess he saw the look on my face and decided to let me in.

I had no clue what any of those machines were or how to use them. But I jumped on to the elliptical trainer and started moving my feet and arms as fast as I could go. In about 60 seconds I thought I was going to die. That was really, scary for a first timer at the gym. My legs burned like mad and I thought that was a sign that I was not supposed to exercise, that I was too heavy to exercise. It was not a fun experience for me.

The gym manager approached me and told me it was normal to feel that way as a newbie. He told me I attacked the elliptical with way too much force and I needed to slow down and pace myself. He suggested that I do one more minute each day until I got up to 30 minutes. *Could it be that simple?* Yup, it was. By adding just one more minute each day, I was able to work out on the elliptical for 30 minutes within 30 days. I felt triumphant. Like I had run a marathon. Cue the *Rocky* theme song in my head! I did it. Something I had so dreaded in the past had become a fun and challenging way to lose weight. Awesome!

The National Weight Control Registry

The National Weight Control Registry is an ongoing research project studying obesity and weight loss. It keeps statistics on people who have lost a significant amount of weight. They regularly survey their membership about lifestyle habits, food choices, and weight-loss maintenance.

The National Weight Control Registry research study includes people 18 years or older who have lost at least 30 pounds and kept it off for at least one year. There are currently over 10,000 members enrolled in the study, making it perhaps the largest study of weight-loss ever conducted. Members complete annual questionnaires about their current weight, diet, and exercise habits, and share behavioral strategies for weight loss maintenance. I am a member of this research project and have participated in their study by completing detailed surveys about my daily habits.

You may find it interesting to know about the people who have enrolled in the registry thus far.

- 80% of people in the registry are women and 20% are men.

- The "average" woman is 45 years of age and currently weighs 145 pounds, while the "average" man is 49 years of age and currently weighs 190 pounds.
- Registry members have lost an average of 66 pounds and kept them off for 5.5 years.
- These averages, however, hide a lot of diversity:
  - Weight losses have ranged from 30 to 300 pounds.
  - Duration of successful weight loss has ranged from one year to 66 years!
  - Some have lost the weight rapidly, while others have lost weight very slowly – over as many as 14 years.
- We have also started to learn about how the weight-loss was accomplished: 45% of registry participants lost the weight on their own and the other 55% lost weight with the help of some type of program.
- 98% of Registry participants report that they modified their food intake in some way to lose weight.
- 94% increased their physical activity, with the most frequently reported form of activity being walking.
- There is variety in how Registry members keep the weight off. Most report continuing to maintain a low-calorie, low-fat diet and doing high levels of activity.
  - 78% eat breakfast every day.
  - 62% watch less than ten hours of TV per week.
  - 90% exercise, on average, about one hour per day.

Keeping a Food Diary

The National Weight Control Registry cites keeping a food diary as one of the most effective tools for weight loss and management.

Keeping a food diary is something I am firmly committed to and that I teach all my clients to do in a way that suits them.

In using a food diary, the goal isn't to turn you into a walking encyclopedia of nutrition, but merely to make you *aware* of the nutritional value of your foods.

For example, we've heard that eating a handful of almonds daily is a good thing. But how much, exactly, is this "handful of almonds"? My handful is about 24 almonds, but my husband's handful is easily twice that. Using a food diary will require you to weigh and measure your food. By doing this, it will become instantly apparent if portion size is your issue, like if you discover that your "handful of almonds" is half a cup. Or that, instead of a portion for you being a reasonable 100 calories, you're actually eating 275. That may not seem like much of a difference, but it will definitely add up over time.

It took a lot of refining over time to arrive at what works for me for steadily losing weight and keeping it off. My food choices don't have to be yours. You can lose weight and maintain your weight with a list of entirely different foods than I choose.

Another great reason to keep a food diary is because it makes you stop and think about your choices *before* you eat, because you know you have to record some information about it before you eat it.

Keeping a food diary is about accountability without judgment, which is great.

And this type of knowledge really is powerful.

You Can't Make a Good Decision without the Facts

I take the opposite approach from diet counselors who look to restrict food choices. Most give you a list of foods to eat and send you off to figure out what that stuff is, where to buy it, and how to cook it. Then, after trying your best to switch from burgers and fries to quinoa and a kale salad, you show up in their office the following month and they wag their finger in judgment over the outcome. That is so unfair.

I can remember showing my steno pad food diary to my counselor one visit when she saw that I'd had two spare ribs at a barbeque. She stood up and said, "You will never eat ribs again." I never went back to see her after that humiliation. And I think of her every time I enjoy eating ribs!

When you commit to keeping a totally honest and complete food diary, you will learn that not everything you're eating is bad or needs to be eliminated. A change in portion size or frequency may be all that is necessary. This has come as a great relief to many of my clients. I don't want to put my clients on a diet. And I don't want you to be hungry or to feel deprived. That always backfires. I want you to look forward to enjoying all the things that are currently working well – and only change what's not working.

Sometimes It's about Your Beverage Choices

It comes as a great surprise to many women when their food diary reveals that it isn't their food that's causing their problem, but instead it is what they are drinking. I'm not talking about alcohol, which can be an issue for some. I'm talking about fruit juices and sugary coffee beverages. Those can really sneak up on you, especially for people who think that juice *must* be healthy, because it's made from fruit. You don't need to drink fruit juice, which often contains more than fruit. You are much better off eating the fruit itself. Juicing is, in my experience with myself and my clients, a waste of time and money and will not help you lose weight. In fact, it can be the cause of weight gain. I don't recommend juicing, but if you like it and want to continue, then put your juice into your food diary and see what impact it has on your total calorie and sugar allotment for the day, and then make the necessary adjustments to fit it in. It's your program and you make the choices. I want you to have all the facts you need to make the best possible decisions for your circumstances.

Meet Paula

Paula is a 48-year-old mother of three who works full-time at a desk job. She has 100 pounds to lose. She sits for most of the day, with a big cup of orange juice on her desk.

On her first visit with me, she told me that she eats pretty well but can't seem to lose any weight. She never drinks sodas – only orange juice, lemonade, and just one vanilla latte per day.

After three days of keeping a food diary, Paula came into my office and reported that she had been stunned to learn that she was drinking about 1300 calories each day, along with over 249 grams of sugar, just in her beverages. That's equivalent to 62 teaspoons, or one-and-one-third cups of sugar per day!

Take a look at these numbers in just these three beverages. Her morning latte has 380 calories with 49 grams of sugar in it. That's all the sugar she needs in an entire day and she drank it for breakfast.

Paula's other go to drink was orange juice and could easily consume a quart or more of it throughout the morning while she worked at her desk. That seemingly "healthy" choice came with 440 calories and another 88 grams of sugar. This is twice the amount of sugar she needed in a day.

And then there is her lemonade, which she realized was a treat but also thought that drinking 32 ounces of it a day was better than drinking soda. Well, I'm sorry to say, it's not. Her lemonade added another 480 calories to her day and a whopping 112 grams of sugar. This is close to three times her limit for the day.

Any one of these beverages was too much and she regularly consumed all three. These three beverages needed to be addressed.

We looked at the math and I suggested that if she would swap the sweetened latte for a skinny version, swap out the orange juice for an actual orange, and change the lemonade for water with a squeeze of fresh lemon in it, she could lose two pounds a week without changing anything else about her food choices! It was tough convincing her it would work, and we did it in stages, but once we weaned her off those three beverages, she lost 100 pounds in about 16 months. Her blood pressure is now normal and she is no longer pre-diabetic. *All she did was change her beverage choices.*

I would not have been able to demonstrate that to her without the benefit of a food diary. In many cases, my clients saw dramatic weight loss by changing only one or two items that were contributing a disproportional amount of calories, and which were discovered by keeping a food diary.

Meet Tom

Tom is six feet tall and weighs 300 pounds. He heard that nuts are a good snack – "a hand full of almonds three or four times a day" is how he described the recommendation he'd heard. On one visit, I had a big bowl of almonds waiting for him and asked Tom to grab "a handful" to show me how much he was eating. His handful was equal to one-third cup, so three or four of those handfuls equated cup or more of almonds. That was way too much fat for him to be snacking on, considering all the other foods he was eating regularly.

We came up with a trail mix for Tom that included his favorite almonds, along with some lower-calorie foods, like puffed rice, toasted oats, dried cranberries, and a few other things. I showed him how much to eat three or four times a day, and soon he was on his way to losing over 40 pounds. *Nothing else changed about his diet*, which was far from perfect. But making the trail mix change was the best he could do given his circumstances. He was then able to get off his blood pressure medications and he is no longer pre-diabetic.

There's an App for That

Although keeping a food diary may seem restrictive, at first, my clients learn that it gives them the freedom to juggle their foods in a way that works best for them.

My advice for keeping a food diary is to find an app to download to your phone. If you use one of the many free websites or apps to keep your food diary, you will gain a very clear understanding of the nutritional value of everything you eat. You will know exactly what you're eating.

My current favorite app is My Fitness Pal. Use that one or another app or system and keep track of what you're eating for a week. Don't put yourself on a diet or try to change your food choices to impress me or anyone else. Just be yourself and do what you do and record everything you eat or drink in a day. The app will tally up all the calories and nutrients. Then review it at the end of the week and you will start to see where your problem is coming from. Adjusting to achieve weight loss will take some trial and error, but that's where the program in this book can help.

Closing the gap between what you are currently eating and what you actually need to eat and do in order to lose weight in a healthy way is critically important to this process. It is the framework of your plan and it will help to guide your daily food choices.

Create a Plan

Do you know the expression *plan the work then work the plan*? Maybe you've heard this one: *No one plans to fail; instead we fail to plan.* We plan for work. We plan our vacations. We plan for our kids, our husbands, the holidays, etc.

We seem to plan for everything except ourselves.

Why? Women typically put their needs last, behind everyone else's needs. So how can you be all that you have the potential to be if you are sleep deprived, feeling anxious because your clothes don't fit, are in pain, or – even worse – are numbing your pain with food or alcohol?

Putting your own self-care first is a big part of your responsibility to those who depend on you.

You're Worth It

It won't take you more than one hour a day to do the things you need to do to take good care of yourself. Considering all that you do and the level of responsibility you carry, an hour a day isn't too much to ask for yourself.

The thing I've found most interesting is that once I wrote out my self-care plan and began to implement it, I actually had more time than less. It seems counter-intuitive, doesn't it? When I took the time to build a plan, I no longer needed to spend time every day wondering what was going to be for dinner, when I could fit in my exercise, or how I was going meet a project deadline. I was confident in the plan I'd laid out for myself and so I only needed to execute each task, and the time to observe the value of the task I had taken.

Once a task made it to my calendar it was non-negotiable.

Identify Your Strengths

We need be brutally honest and put all your cards on the table. Let's figure out what we're working with regarding how you spend your time and attention.

What do you most enjoy doing? Be honest. What do you lose track of time doing? Can you remember when you were so engrossed in something that time stood still? Or maybe time flew by so fast you realized that what felt like minutes was really hours passing. There are tasks you do a lot because you like to. Because of this, you're good at them, you're confident about your ability to do them, and you can manage any obstacle that comes along. Over time you've become an expert and the effort involved in completing these tasks is minimal and doing those tasks is enjoyable.

These tasks are your strengths.

Make a list. You may be surprised at what you discover.

Learn from Your Weaknesses

There are also things you dread doing. There are certain situations or people you avoid and who you're uncomfortable around. You're not confident in those circumstances or with those people, and you feel awkward.

Understanding where those feeling come from can help you overcome your weaknesses. For now, I just want you to acknowledge them. This is where we need to put some focus. Acknowledge that you haven't been successful in the past, but also know that you can learn to use these characteristics in your favor as well. Add these to your list of strengths in a separate column.

Here's an example. I knew I had a problem eating out in restaurants, so I put that on my list of weaknesses. I'd become easily distracted by the conversation and lose track of how much bread I was eating. I knew I would have to eventually learn how to control myself in that situation, because I wanted to be able to go out to dinner with friends. Simply being aware of my weakness in that situation allowed me to be more alert at dinners with friends. I went in thinking, *Yes, this is going to be challenging for me, but I'm aware now and can look for ways to take control.*

Use Both Strengths and Weaknesses to Your Advantage

Look at your lists. What are your strengths and weaknesses? Be honest. This is just between you and you. Are you a really good planner and a great cook? Do you hate to exercise? Do you rarely drink water?

Review your list and then let's use these findings to work with your old habits and gently realign them with new health goals. Instead of trying to change direction by turning 180 degrees, we'll move just a few degrees at a time.

Don't judge your strengths and also your weaknesses. Just know that they are habits you currently have and use them in combination to get what you want.

Are You a Creature of Habit?

One thing we know for sure – the more you do something, the better you get at it. You do it faster, more efficiently, and with less and less thought, until it becomes a habit. This is a really good thing, for the most part. We are all creatures of habit.

Imagine if you had to *think* about putting one foot in front of the other each time you wanted to walk across the room. Fortunately for most of us, walking is a habit we learned early in life and it now requires very little conscious thought to do.

In the beginning, when you first learned to walk, your new little brain had a difficult time directing your weak, wobbly little legs. At first, even standing up was a big accomplishment. Each step was applauded and you were encouraged to keep going. Each time you fell, you were picked up so you could try again, until you mastered the complex set of actions called *walking* and your brain was able to file them away in the back of your mind.

There was never any question that you'd keep trying until you were walking. No one saw you fall and said, "Oh leave her there. She'll never be able to walk. This is too hard to watch. What's the point?" Instead, you kept working toward that goal, and now you can walk. Now thoughts about putting one foot in front of the other never seem to come up. But that's only because you've done it a bazillion times, so you're really efficient at it. The thoughts are still running in the background, like the operating system on your computer. You don't notice and it doesn't take much effort, though, because it's become a habit.

We tend to take some of our habits for granted because they require so little conscious effort.

You Can Build Good Habits as Easily as You Build Bad Ones

This same concept of habit formation works equally as well with bad habits as with good ones. The more you practice, the better you get. You got really efficient at mastering the skill of walking at an early age and then you learned to drive. OMG! How confusing was *that* when you had to look ahead, check the side in the mirrors, *and* know which pedals to push, all at once? Do you remember your first time behind the wheel? I do. It was scary and thrilling at the same time, but it took every ounce of focus and concentration I had to move that 1969 Red Buick Skylark down my street. It was exhausting. And now? I sometimes wonder how I got to my destination, because driving is such an efficient process after all these years of practice, that I was able to think about something else altogether while I was doing it.

My point is simply that if you continue to do the same thing over and over it will become a habit. Whether it's a good thing or a bad thing it will become effortless. I choose to spend my time developing habits that serve me by taking me closer to my goals. The more I do them the easier it gets.

Understanding my habits and putting them to work for me was the key to my weight loss success. Habits make life easy – sometimes, as long as they are directed toward your goal. Separating the good habits you have from the bad ones requires self-reflection and honesty with yourself. Many times, we don't see our bad habits as easily as someone else will. It pays to have a neutral third party to talk with who can help you identify your blind spots and whose opinion and knowledge you trust.

Where Are Your Habits Pulling You?

Can you observe a habit in action? Imagine you're at the top of a ski slope that you've been skiing down over and over all day. There are ruts in the snow and you can stick your skis into them and make it down the hill to the same place at the bottom every time, with your eyes closed, after doing it all day. Just place your skis in the grooves and away you go.

But imagine if you wanted to end up at a different place at the bottom of the hill. You're going to have to point your skis in a different direction at the top of the hill in order to end up at your new destination down below. And those helpful ruts won't be there.

Not only that, but a minor shift in your direction will create a major change in your destination. At first, your skis will want to find those old ruts in the snow. But just a slight nudge to the left or right will take you to a completely different destination.

It's the same way with your food habits.

Let's identify those old habits, strengths, and weaknesses, then nudge them slightly so you will arrive at new destination. Over time, you will create new ruts in the snow and new pathways in your brain that are the new healthy habits you seek.

Make Room in Your Life for Healthy Habits

There came a time in my life when I wanted to move to a new house. Now, keep in mind that I live in a great area where people pay lots of money to go on vacation, especially in the summers. I love living on Long Island, for so many reasons. I soon realized my new-house search really wasn't about finding a new climate to live in (going to Florida is the norm around here after a certain age). I wasn't looking for a bigger house or looking to downsize necessarily, either. My neighbors are fine; my commute to work is a breeze; my house is in great repair – so what was up with the desire to move?

It finally occurred to me that I really didn't want to leave my current home as much as I wanted less stuff in my home. I wanted the newness that came from only having the stuff that was useful to me, without all the other stuff in my closets and attic. If I bought another home, I'd want it to be just like the one I was already living in, so, instead, I put myself through the process of editing the stuff I was living with.

I wanted to move out of my old house and back into the same house, but with only the stuff that was relevant to my current life and that would support my current lifestyle.

With my commitment to only keep was serving me, I methodically went through every closet, drawer, garage, attic, and tool shed, with my husband's help. We focused on one closet or area of the garage per weekend and only worked for one hour. Week after week, we kept doing that, and soon there was less and less stuff clogging my house and my mind.

Having less stuff and having only the things I really wanted seemed to make my life easier and reduced my stress level. I could easily find whatever I was looking for, instead of running out to buy another of something that was buried in the garage. Having less stuff also meant that I had less to take care of, store, and maintain.

When it comes to finding room in your life for the healthy habits I'm asking you to adopt, you'll need to make room for them in your life by eliminating those habits that are not serving you. Just like cleaning out a closet.

Are You Ready to Make a Change?

There is a process for making changes that I'd like to discuss here. Many times women will come to me before they are really ready to commit and they stick with me for a few weeks, sort of applying themselves but not fully committed to doing the work that it takes to make permanent changes and create new healthy habits. This is okay, really. It's all part of the decision-making process. I have found with these clients that when they do come back to me later, they are really ready and are successful and efficient in getting the job done.

In order for you to truly conquer this weight mystery, you need to create a lifestyle of healthy habits that support your goal. You cannot have one foot in your old lifestyle and one in your new lifestyle that you want and expect permanent results. You've got to go all in. But you don't need to become a gym rat to have a healthy body.

The Four Stages of Change

In the beginning stage of behavior change we see people in *pre-contemplation*. Using exercise as an example, someone in pre-contemplation would be sedentary and not even considering exercising. They do not see exercise as relevant in their lives and may even argue with the need for or importance of physical activity. I remained in this stage for most of my life.

Contemplation follows. In this stage, people are still sedentary, but they are starting to consider the value of regular exercise. They have begun to consider being active, but are not yet doing anything. This is the stage where you mentally "try on" an idea, and often discard many, until you actually try something new. Getting stuck here is common, especially if you're someone who is afraid of making a mistake.

Then comes *preparation.* In this stage, people will get some exercise here and there as they mentally and physically prepare to adopt an exercise program. Activity during this stage will be erratic and inconsistent. But this is still progress. During this phase, many people will get to the gym once or twice a week, but if they don't see movement on the scale, they are ready to give up, which they do – until they get angry at themselves for giving up and give it yet another try. This pattern is typical of yo-yo dieters.

Action is the phase when people are engaging in regular exercise but have been doing it for less than six months. This is a fun stage to be in because your body is getting used to the regular exercise and the benefits are starting to show in different areas of your life. You start to become a believer. By this point, you are ready to commit and leave your old lifestyle behind. However, the behaviors are still relatively new to you and you can easily be distracted.

Finally, the *maintenance* stage of behavior change comes when you have been taking consistent action for more than six months.

This is when you're on fire. There is no way that you are going to spend another day living with unhealthy exercise habits. You are committed to getting a reasonable amount of appropriate exercise. That is simply *what you do*. This is how you roll. Exercising is no big deal. Exercising fits nicely into your life. You'd miss it if you couldn't do it. You don't feel guilty pressure about it.

This is the place to be!

To Do:

Get yourself a calendar program. Get one you like or use a spreadsheet for this experiment. Start with a blank calendar and pencil in your priorities. No more making to do lists or promising that you'll start on Monday. Instead, put whatever you intend to do on your calendar. Start today with one little thing that is going to be different. Try your new habit for four days and then decide if you're going to keep doing it. If it makes it on to your usual, permanent calendar, then it is non-negotiable. It's like an appointment with your boss. There's no way you'd miss it. I started doing this process with sleep. I know I function best with seven hours of sleep and I wanted to be in my office by 9:00 a.m. So I had to be in bed by 10:30, no exceptions. I put that in my regular calendar and then did it.

Make an honest list of your strengths and weaknesses.

Chapter 5
Food

You probably thought food would have come up before Chapter 5 in a book to help you lose weight. It absolutely is a very important element, but it also needs to be put into proper perspective.

Let me give you the bottom line: You're overweight because you've eaten more calories than you've burned over a period of time. That's it. And the key to bringing you back to your ideal weight is to burn those extra calories over time.

But you also know that this process is so much more than eating less of this or that, so let's look at what you need to know about your food choices. In later chapters, we'll move on to why this concept is so easy to comprehend, yet seemingly impossible to apply.

"Do I Have to Give up All My Favorite Foods?"

Here's my promise: You *do not* have to change everything about what you eat to lose weight permanently. It's possible there are a just a few foods which arc mostly responsible for your excess weight. You never have to starve yourself; you don't have to give up all the foods you like; you don't have to cut out all of any food group, like fats or carbs; and you don't have to drink shakes. Also, everything you need to eat can be purchased at any supermarket, and you don't need to spend hours cooking, shopping, and prepping.

Food was way too important to me to ever think I could happily lose weight and keep it off. I'm a foodie and I love to cook. But here's the thing that's so confounding to a lot of us: I got to be 320 pounds by eating really delicious, good, healthy food. I didn't pig out on candy, cookies, soda, or chips. The interviewer from *People* asked me if I ever ate a whole pizza or a box of waffles. "Do you keep donuts in your bedroom?" No, no, and no. I was only interested in quality foods that I found on fine restaurant menus or cooked at home with the best ingredients. I grew up in my Italian grandmother's kitchen and remember sitting on two phone books so I could reach the table as I helped her close the homemade raviolis. With food, cooking or entertaining a big part of my life, you know I wasn't going to be happy eating rice cakes and celery sticks for two years in order to lose weight.

Rules to Live By

For me, there are a few rules that always apply to my food. You get to write your own list of rules, which may be very different from mine. As long as your rules are effective and not harmful, they're your choice. It doesn't matter if they work for anyone else but you.

Here are my rules:

- My food must always be delicious, healthy, fresh, and simply prepared.
- If I don't like it, I'm not eating it, even if it's good for me.
- I don't want to commit more than 30 minutes to dinner prep on a work night.

In order to meet those criteria, I had to take a hard look at what I was eating, and be willing to open my mind to new ideas, ingredients, or cooking methods. I got to work in the kitchen and experimented – a lot. I want to take a moment to thank my husband and my office mates for their kind help as taste testers. They were fearless!

No fake foods or diet versions for me. I will not accept anything that doesn't taste delicious, look great, and fit within my current nutritional goals. I eat delicious food every day. And I always know there's another delicious meal waiting for me later that day or the next day.

What's in Your Fridge?

People always ask me the same two questions: "What do you eat every day?" and "Will you write a meal plan for me?" The answer to the first question is that I eat simple, unfussy, recognizable, delicious foods that I record daily in my food diary. Will I write a meal plan for you? Absolutely not, and I'll tell you why. I don't know you. I don't know what you like to eat, what your heritage is, how much you like to cook, how much time you have to cook, whether you have kids or not, whether you eat at home or prefer to go out? Only you know those things.

That is why keeping an unguided food diary is your starting point. It allows us to carve away what is not working and rebalance your choices so they take you closer to your goal. I'd rather teach you to fish so you can feed yourself for a life time.

My first food diary entries included large quantities of empty-calorie carbs, like buttered bagels or pancakes and maple syrup for breakfast. Lunch was a deli sandwich of turkey and cheese with mayo and a bag of chips. Dinner could be three slices of pizza and a diet soda. Don't ask me why I ate like that, but I insisted on diet soda and then ice cream for a late night snack. That was an improvement for me, because previously there would have been two or three donuts eaten in the conference room at work and then also a snack I grabbed on my way to catch my train home. Looking back, I realize now how fortunate I am to not have developed major heart health issues.

My eating evolution was slow and deliberate. Since I didn't know what I was doing, I started with cutting the serving sizes of the same foods I'd been eating – and my weight began to drop.

Food Facts

I want to give you just the very basic info and the simplest tools so you make healthy choices when you are faced with a food decision, something that occurs about 300 times a day. I want you to always enjoy your food – and then move on with your day. No guilt. No regrets. Don't focus on what to avoid. Instead, let's find foods you love that work toward your goal.

Did you know that calories only come from three macronutrient sources? Those are carbs, fats, and proteins. That's it. There are no calories in fiber or sodium, and things without gluten still have calories. Good fats and bad fats are all still fats.

It's that simple.

If you'll allow me a moment on my soap box, I'll tell you that I am appalled at how much time and money is spent by big business to try to confuse consumers into thinking that something is healthy by using words like *gluten-free*, *natural*, *low-sugar*, or *low-fat*. Don't believe anything you read on the front of a package. It's just marketing hype created to sell more products – smoke and mirrors. The only truth on a package is in the nutrition label, so let's start there.

Nutrition Facts
Serving Size 3 oz. (85g)
Serving Per Container 2

Amount Per Serving

Calories 200	Calories from Fat 120

	% Daily Value*
Total Fat 15g	**20 %**
Saturated Fat 5g	**28 %**
Trans Fat 3g	
Cholesterol 30mg	**10 %**
Sodium 650mg	**28 %**
Total Carbohydrate 30g	**10 %**
Dietary Fiber 0g	**0 %**
Sugars 5g	
Protein 5g	

Vitamin A 5%	•	Vitamin C 2%
Calcium 15%	•	Iron 5%

*Percent Daily Values are based on a 2,000 calorie diet. Your Daily Values may be higher or lower depending on your calorie needs.

	Calories	2,000	2,500
Total Fat	Less than	65g	80g
Sat Fat	Less than	20g	25g
Cholesterol	Less than	300mg	300mg
Sodium	Less than	2,400mg	2,400mg
Total Carbonhydrate		300mg	375mg
Dietary Fiber		25g	30g

This is a look at the new nutrition label approved by the FDA:

The nutrition label is important information that is often overlooked when teaching children about what to eat. Most "diet" programs hope you never read the nutrition label on the packages of the food they require you to buy from them. They'd rather you be fooled by the pretty pictures on the front of the package or by the images of the 23-year-old fitness model who doesn't eat this stuff. She was paid a bunch of money to have her picture taken and she makes a living doing just that. It's no wonder she looks great – she gets paid to look great. This is so deceptive. Forget all the stuff you see on the package and believe only what's in that black and white box called "Nutrition Facts." This should be required learning in all of our schools.

Macro Nutrients

We need to eat a particular amount of each macro nutrient based on our body's needs and goals. The three macro nutrient groups are carbohydrates, fats, and proteins. As we discussed before, these are our only sources of calories. It is important to get an adequate supply of our foods from each group. I want you to have a basic understanding of the role, sources, and value of each of the macro nutrients. You will learn much about this from a careful review of your food journal. Eventually this information will become second nature to you.

Carbs

Carbohydrates are organic compounds found in our food in the form of starch and sugar. Carbs have four calories per gram and they typically equate to 50% of the daily calorie allotment. All sugars are carbs, but not all carbs are sugar. I'll show you more about this if you do a food journal with me.

Carbohydrates are the main source of energy for our bodies. Although carbohydrates may be vilified by trendy diets, they should be consumed on a daily basis. Carbohydrates are essential to our well-being, to our brain function, and to the functioning of many cells within our bodies. Never ever give up all your carbs in an effort to lose weight, please. It's not healthy.

"Where Do Carbs Come From?"

Here's a general rule: If it used to be a plant, it's a carb. Easy, right? Carbs are found in grains, fruits, vegetables, and beans. The only exception to this rule is that carbs are also found in dairy foods.

Carbohydrates can be really good and healthy or contain nothing but empty calories. Choose carbohydrates that come from whole grains and from whole, fresh (not dried or canned) fruits and vegetables. These are typically called *good carbs* (for good reason). If you can still recognize what it was when it was growing, it's a good carb. If you have no idea what it comes from, then stay away.

Processed foods that contain added sugars – such as cookies, candy, bottled salad dressings and sauces, fruit juices, and sodas – also contain carbs, but in a refined form. Refined carbohydrates are empty calories and should be minimized; they contribute nothing to your long-term wellness and can keep you going back for more, as they truly are addictive. Our brains react to refined sugar in a way that's similar to how it responds to another white powder: cocaine.

So many of my clients come in proudly announcing that they are giving up carbs in order to lose weight. Please wait before you declare all carbs off-limits! Carbs are necessary and not evil at all.

"How Many Carbs Should I Eat?"

Since carbohydrates are the body's main source of energy, you need about 50% to 55% of your total daily caloric intake from carbs. That seems like a lot for my clients who have been beaten into submission by the Atkins craze. For the average woman, that equals to 1000 calories, or 250 grams of carbs a day!

A piece of fruit or a slice of bread contains 15 grams of carbs, while a serving of vegetables typically contains 5 grams of carbs. But grab a sweetened latte and a muffin on the way to work and you may use up most of your daily carb allotment before noon. Even more shocking is when you see how much sugar is in that smoothie they sell at the gym. Yikes! Once I did the math, I realized why those smoothie bars exist in gyms. It's to make sure you never lose a pound so you keep coming back.

To Do

> **Learn which and how much carbs work for you and how to enjoy them without guilt.**

Fats

According to the American Heart Association, dietary fats perform a necessary role in providing your body with energy and to support cell growth. They also help protect your organs and help keep your body warm. Fats help your body to absorb some nutrients and produce important hormones, too. Your body definitely needs dietary fat to function well.

Not all fats are good for you. We've heard a lot about good fats and bad fats, and figuring out which is which can be confusing. Without giving you too much information, I want you to remember that there are four types of fats we consume in our diets. These are the four major dietary fats in the foods we eat:

1. saturated fats
2. trans fats
3. monounsaturated fats
4. polyunsaturated fats

The four types have different chemical structures and physical properties. The bad fats are the saturated and trans fats, and they tend to be more solid at room temperature (like a stick of butter), while the better fats – monounsaturated and polyunsaturated fats – tend to be more liquid at room temperature (like liquid vegetable oil).

Fats can also have different effects on the cholesterol levels in your body. The bad fats (saturated fats and trans fats) raise bad cholesterol (LDL) levels in your blood. Monounsaturated fats and polyunsaturated fats can lower bad cholesterol levels, and are beneficial when consumed as part of a healthy dietary pattern.

"Where Do Good Fats Come From?"

Fats come from both plant and animal sources. We want to go with the plant fats and avoid the animal fats. So when you think good fats, think avocado, nuts, olive oil. Salmon is an exception to the plant fat rule.

"How Much Fat Do I Need in a Day?"

Dietary fats have nine calories per gram and can vary from 20-35% of your total calorie consumption for the day.

The bottom line is that eating foods with fat is definitely part of a healthy diet. Just remember to choose foods that provide good fats. Doing so means that your diet will be low in both saturated fats and trans fats.

Proteins

Proteins function as building blocks for bones, muscles, cartilage, skin, blood, enzymes, hormones, and vitamins. They play a vital role in the function of the nervous system, aid in the formation of red blood cells, and help build tissues. Protein is essential to maintaining the body's systems and functions.

Sources of protein include both animal and plant foods, but if you follow a vegetarian or vegan diet, you are likely still able to eat adequate amounts of complete proteins solely from plant sources. Eating a diet that includes a variety of foods from all food groups will allow you to get the amount of protein necessary for your body to build muscle and maintain organs.

"Where Does Protein Come From?"

Proteins are either manufactured by our cells or are found in our diets. Protein sources include animal products such as meat, poultry, fish, eggs, and dairy. Protein can also come from plant sources such as nuts, seeds, whole grains, and beans. My favorite clean, lean proteins are fish of any type, egg whites, Greek non-fat plain yogurt, turkey, chicken breasts, and pork tenderloin.

"How Much Protein Do I Need?"

Proteins have four calories per gram and typically vary from 20-30% of your daily total. Protein intake needs change throughout a person's lifecycle, but for the most part, we can determine our needs using a simple equation (more about this later). Our protein needs can be met easily throughout the day by including a source of protein at each meal or snack.

"Can I Eat Too Much Protein?"

Excess protein in the diet can have side effects when paired with a low-carbohydrate intake. This may lead to dehydration, fatigue, and bad breath. When fruits and vegetables are under-consumed and replaced with excess protein, it can put a strain on the heart and lead to vitamin and mineral deficiencies. Moderate amounts of protein, along with a diet rich in nutrient-dense foods – such as fruits, vegetables, and whole grains –make for a well-rounded eating pattern that supports optimal health.

"What about Alcohol?"

Alcohol has seven calories per gram and zero nutritional value but does not need to be completely eliminated – once you understand how to fit it in. Alcohol is not off-limits in my program as long as you make an informed decision and record it in your food diary. Yes, you can enjoy wine with dinner or a drink with friends.

Let's Go to the Supermarket

I've taken many clients on a tour of a supermarket, because they simply had never been taught how to shop for food. There's nothing to be ashamed of here, so let's get down to basics.

As a busy person who has so little time for herself, you need to get in and out of the grocery store quickly, and this method makes shopping really fast. Here it is: *Stay out of the middle of the store.* Seriously, everything you need to live a healthy life is on the perimeter. Notice how little packaging and labeling there is on the foods around the perimeter. It is where the freshest, simplest, unfussiest foods are. It's really easy to zip around the perimeter, and then you're done.

Once you start down the aisles, you get sucked into the marketing haze of pretty packaging and misleading labels. There are entire aisles I never visit. Soda? Chips? No. Cookies, crackers, and candy? No. The squishy breads aisle? Sorry, no. Canned foods? Nope, not ever. There are no foods in those aisles that I feel are worth the calories, and they aren't tempting or calling me. They just have no purpose in my life. No drama. How much time did I just take off your shopping trips?

"How Much Can I Eat and Still Lose Weight?"

This question comes up a lot. Most people have no idea what weight is right for them. There is a general guideline for figuring out what weight you need to achieve to maintain a healthy body weight. You can request a free tool kit from my website that will help you determine your total caloric needs for a day: www.debbielazinsky.com.

But this is not about calories alone. As any experienced dieter knows, the story does not end with "calories in vs. calories out." If only it were that simple. The quality and source of your calories are also of utmost importance. Specifically, you can eat the right number of calories and still be poorly nourished if the source of those calories is out of balance with your needs.

Do the Math

Let's start with figuring out the total number of calories you need to consume in a day by following this example. (If you need help figuring your goal weight or any of the numbers appropriate for you, send an email with "DO THE MATH" in the subject line to me at debbie@debbielazinsky.com.)

For this example, the goal weight is 140 pounds.

1. For a sedentary lifestyle, multiply the goal weight (140) by 12 = 1680 calories.
2. For an active lifestyle, multiply the result of step 1 (1680) by 1.2 = 2016 calories.

3. For a very active lifestyle, multiply the result of step 1 (1680) by 1.3 = 2184 calories.

Simple, right? The result of the math will be an estimate. If you want to know precisely what your body needs, using a fitness tracker like a FITBIT is a great way to see what you're burning.

This is a great equation to use for maintenance and general weight loss.

How to Calculate Your Macronutrients

Once you have your daily calorie number from the equation above, you are ready to break it down into the amounts of carbs, fats, and proteins required to reach your goal.

This calculation will depend on your goals. For example, for fat loss in a healthy individual, I may recommend a proportion of 50% carbs, 25 % fat, and 25 % proteins.

Let's look at an example, using 1680 daily calories:

Carbs. Divide your daily calorie goal by two – this equals the total number of calories per day to allocate to carbs. In our example, that's 840 calories. Then divide that result by four for the number of carb grams per day that you need. In this example, that would be 210 grams of carbs daily.

Proteins. Divide your daily calorie goal by four – this equals the total number of calories per day to allocate to proteins. In our example, that's 420 calories. Divide that result by four. This equals the number of protein grams you would need daily. In this example, that's 105.

Fats. Divide your daily calorie goal by four – this equals 420 in our example. Then divide 420 by nine to get the number of fat grams you need daily. In this example, that's 47.

To Do

> **Use a food journal to track your foods eaten against your goal.**
> Once you have your daily calories and macronutrient numbers,
> use a food journal app to track your foods eaten against your
> goals to see how close you are to eating a healthy balanced diet.

"What's on Your Top 40 List?"

When I ask a client why they eat a certain way or hold a certain belief about food, many of them respond the same way: "I don't know. I've always eaten that way." Nooooooo – it wasn't always that way. You were not born with the natural instinct to order béarnaise sauce on your filet mignon. You *learned* to love it because you tried it once, it tasted good, and you remembered that new, awesome taste sensation, filing it away under "GET MORE SOON." These foods are a pure joy to eat. And those random acts of desire are what formed the basis for your Top 40.

Most people eat, on average, about 40 different foods on a regular basis. I have analyzed thousands of food diaries and it is surprising how consistent this number is. Once you start to ask yourself *why* you are eating those foods, you become naturally more selective in what goes into your Top 40.

Fuel or Fun

I want you to break down your Top 40 into two distinct groups: fuel or fun. All your food should taste good and look appealing to you. I never want you to suffer through eating things that are "good for you" if you don't like them. Stop that right now! Foods you define as fuel foods should provide your body with the nourishment it needs to do the things you want to do. Do they leave you feeling good, energized, in control, and happy with yourself? If so, they deserve to be on your fuel foods list.

It's kind of ironic to think of how I used to scrutinize any medication that was prescribed for me, even if I only had to take it for a week, to see if it might contain something I didn't want to ingest, and yet I spent the better part of 50 years making horrible food choices and not thinking twice about it.

Fun Foods

About 10% to 20% of my calories are allocated to food that just tastes good. This could be kale or brownies or wine. I don't really care, as long as they bring me pure joy. I eat them because I want to. I don't apologize for it, I don't hide it from my husband, and I never feel guilty about it. Anything goes, as long as it consumes no more than 20% of my calorie goal for that day.

Using your food diary is especially important for learning how to manage this concept. When 80% to 90% of what you're eating on a regular basis is truly fuel for your body, then allow yourself the pure indulgence of fun foods 10 to 20% of the time.

Size Does Matter

Dr. Barbara J. Rolls' book *The Volumetrics Weight Control Plan* taught me a lot about how to satisfy my need for a large volume of food – but with fewer calories. It was surprising to me to learn that we generally eat the same volume of food each day. We humans have developed a skill for deciding how much food is "enough.". This can help you because you can change to eating fewer calories without consuming a smaller volume of food. The key concept at work here is that we generally eat with our eyes first, so we need to pick the foods that will satisfy our eyes as well as our taste and nutritional needs.

"That's All the Food I Need for Now"

I realized, after observing my own reactions to being served in a restaurant, that I had developed a habit of evaluating the volume of food in front of me and instantly deciding if it would be enough. It would drive me crazy when I'd go to dinner with my husband and the waiter would put our plates down in front of us and I'd instantly compare his portion to mine, thinking they decided in the kitchen that I needed to lose weight, so they gave me the smaller piece of steak. I was so convinced that was standard restaurant protocol that I'd have my husband order for me so the waiter wouldn't know if it was his dish or mine until it was at the table. And yet, somehow, they always knew and made my portion smaller than his. Never mind that I would have been more than satisfied had I eaten without judgment the portion I was served. That didn't matter. I had already made up my mind that I was going to be short-changed, singled out, and pre-judged by the kitchen and wait staff. That made me angry and frustrated, which is not conducive to a pleasant dinner out. Of course, the restaurant staff's campaign against me was completely untrue – but I carried that belief around for a long time.

I'm a Volume Eater

Rather than trying to use willpower to help me accept a tiny portion, I acknowledged the fact that I liked to eat larger portions of food. I had a big appetite.

There, I said it. So what?

I was not interested in fighting with myself for the rest of my life – *that* is "dieting." Noticing that I had a habit of comparing my portion sizes was a clue to my discovery that I could "inflate" the volume on my plate by working into my recipes foods that took up a lot of space on the plate but didn't have lots of calories. This concept has served me all these years to maintain my weight and to teach clients how to modify recipes in a way that will allow them to eat the foods they love while losing weight.

Think for a minute about unbuttered, air-popped popcorn. It's nothing but corn and air. There are 100 calories in one cup of popcorn. That's a big volume of food. For comparison, there is the same number of calories in one tablespoon of butter. These two foods are on the opposite ends of the calorie density scale. Popcorn would be on the very low end of the scale, meaning it has lots of volume and few calories; butter is on the other end of the scale because it is calorie-dense, with a large number of calories relative to its small size. The reason popcorn is so filling is because of its air and fiber content.

Water-rich foods are also very satisfying. This is different than drinking water, however, which does quench thirst but will not satisfy hunger. Water-rich foods, like fresh fruits and vegetables, add volume to your dish without adding many calories. For example, adding chopped spinach to your meatloaf recipe cuts down on the calories in the portions served, because spinach will take the place of higher-calorie foods in the recipe, like the ground meat or cheese. Your portion looks the same on the plate, but the actual calorie count is much lower.

Think about adding fresh fruit to your pancakes or lots of raw veggies to your sandwich. When you pay attention to the volume of food you can eat and pick the right foods, you'll never feel deprived. This is a huge hurdle to overcome and is a welcome relief to women who have trained themselves that starvation is the only way to lose weight.

Think about the difference between fresh fruit and dried fruits. Take dried apples, for example: a quarter-cup of dried apple slices have the equivalent amount of calories and sugar as a whole fresh apple. This is because the dried apples no longer contain the water of a fresh apple. The calories and sugars are reduced to a much smaller quarter-cup serving.

Fats are on the opposite end of the calorie-density scale and are the fastest way to add calories to any dish. Fats have more than twice the calories per gram than carbs and proteins.

When you combine these strategies by adding high water content and high fiber foods to your plate while at the same time cutting some of the fat, you'll have a delicious and satisfying meal that fits within your daily calorie budget.

I love the example in Barbara's book about 200 calories of soup and how different the serving size will be depending on how much fat is in the soup. She clearly illustrates that when you choose a soup with less fat you can eat more soup.

Each of these servings of soup has 200 calories:

- 1 cup cream of broccoli with cheese
- 1-1/4 cups New England clam chowder
- 1-3/4 cups chicken with rice
- 2-1/2 cups vegetable with beef broth

As I analyzed the nutritional value of my recipes, I quickly realized that many of my old favorite foods were full of sugar or fat, or lacking in protein or fiber. Learning to add volume to my meals and recipes made all the difference in the world to me.

Lighten Up

I have been very successful at recreating old favorites in healthier versions, so I was able to eat the foods I enjoy and not have to restrict myself to a short list of allowed foods, or survive on lettuce and rice cakes. Not when I could add mushrooms to my meatloaf or make a fruit cobbler instead of pie. Life is too short not to enjoy each meal!

I *love* to modify comfort foods or family traditional recipes to meet my clients' nutritional needs. I'm not willing to compromise on taste and texture, especially with family traditions. That is too important to me to ever let go of. These are the foods we used to celebrate holidays and special occasions. They have come to represent love and good memories and connection to our heritage – and they are generally very high in calories.

There's a family tradition that was on every holiday table at home for as long as I can remember. My father's mother made it. I thought she invented it, but it turns out it's a traditional Italian favorite. It's called *pizza rustica*. It's like a big, savory cheesecake. It's thick with cheese, salami, eggs, and ham and is surrounded by pie crust. It costs a fortune to make and I *love* it. I can remember waiting for it to come out of the oven and then eating piece after piece.

Then, one day, after I had lost my weight and the holiday was coming, I asked my mom for the recipe. OMG. When I did the recipe analysis, I learned that this family favorite was probably responsible for the early deaths by heart attack of both my father and grandfather. It should be classified as a lethal weapon and come with a warning label. But it tasted so good. So I went to work and, after much trial and error, was able to keep the tradition – as well as myself alive – with my lightened up version.

Beware of Portion Distortion

In the beginning, I started out weighing and measuring my foods very carefully. Once I had done it a number of times, I thought I could judge by eye or use a common item as a reference. You know, a reference like a deck of cards is about the size of your protein and a half-cup is about the size of a computer mouse. But here's the problem: Little by little, those referenced portions seemed to grow, over time. So you need to regularly refresh your memory. This was painfully obvious to me when I measured olive oil by the tablespoon after using my "judgement" for weeks. I realized that one tablespoon had somehow grown to two. That may not sound like a big deal until you do the math and realize the compound effect of that small amount of unaccounted for calories.

One tablespoon of olive oil, a good fat, has about 120 calories. So when I was using two and recording just one in my diary, there were 120 calories unaccounted for. Since I have a salad almost every day, that 120 calories could add up to an extra 12 pounds a year. Do that for ten years and, there you go – you now have an extra 120 pounds that just seemed to creep up on you. Most people would realize there was a problem after about ten or 20 pounds and go on a diet, meaning starving, eating weird food, or subjecting themselves to some other form of torture, when all they'd really have to do is go back to one tablespoon of olive oil and the weight would disappear as slowly and naturally as it had appeared.

I don't measure and weigh everything any longer, but I make it a practice to measure all my foods once a week, just to make sure portion distortion isn't setting in. I do this every Monday and call it Measure Up Monday. It's a silly name that helped me to remember until it became a habit.

To Do

Identify your Top 40. Take look at your food diary. What have you eaten over the past month? Are those foods providing fuel for your body? Then they deserve a place on your fuel foods list. But let's not forget about fun foods. Allocate 10% to 20% of your calories to some food on your Top 40 list *just because it tastes good.*

Make a list of things you like to do because they're just fun. Plan to include a little fun in every day. No excuses necessary. This little trick will keep you focused, because you know that there's always room for a little fun.

Get a free copy of some of my comfort food recipes in your free tool kit. Go to www.debbielazinsky.com.

||||||||||||||||||||||||||||||||

Chapter 6

Rest, Repair, and Recharge

etting enough rest through quality sleep is a very important
part of the day. So many of my clients underestimate the value
rest contributes to good health, or they're sleep deprived and
don't realize it. Among other things, while you are sleeping your
body is repairing itself and your brain is recharging

Chronic loss of sleep has been linked to health risks like obesity,
high blood pressure, heart disease, and stroke. It is also likely to cause
daytime drowsiness, irritability, forgetfulness, and an inclination
toward mistakes and accidents. The Center for Disease Control
reports that 35% of Americans fail to get enough sleep.

Rather than trying to catch up on lost sleep over the weekends,
I find that it is much more beneficial to get consistent sleep all week
long. Adequate sleep is toward the top of my priority list. It's a great
new, healthy habit to learn.

Create a Sleep Ritual

Start by planning to go to bed early enough to get seven to eight hours of sleep.

Create a two-hour buffer before actually going to bed during which you start to "power down." During this time, turn off your electronic devices, including the TV, and engage in relaxing activities instead. I love to take a warm lavender bubble bath while reading, sipping chamomile tea, and listening to soft music.

Make sure your bedroom is quiet, dark, and soothing.

Your bed should be comfortable and your pillow and linens fresh and cozy.

Deep Breathing Exercise

This is a great tip to help you fall asleep, but it is also great to help you refocus your attention and bring you into the present moment. I do this when I'm stressed or overwhelmed and every night when my head hits the pillow. Try it yourself. You'll be amazed.

- Get into a comfortable position, in bed for the night.
- Breathe in slowly and deeply through your nose while you count to four. Fill your lungs all the way.
- Hold your breath while you count to five.
- Blow out air like you're blowing out a candle – forcefully through your mouth – as you count to six.
- Repeat for a total of seven times (if you're still awake).

To Do:

Replace your mattress and pillows. When was the last time you replaced your mattress and pillows? Treat yourself to the luxury of high-quality linens.

Look at your daily schedule and pencil in your bedtime.

Chapter 7

"Exercise? Do I Have To?"

The thought of exercise used to cause a knot in my stomach. I dreaded it, I wasn't good at it, I hated to sweat, and I would be totally freaked out to be seen in stretchy workout clothes. The reasons I completely avoided the topic were endless.

What's Holding You Back?

What I came to realize was that fear was holding me back. All of the fears that drove my desire to eat were the same fears that kept me from exercising. That was a startling revelation I had when I began to examine why I avoided doing certain things.

Fear had a grip on my life. I was afraid of being ridiculed at the gym for being so overweight, so I'd skip the gym and soothe myself with chocolate chip cookies. Talk about a double whammy:

not exercising and eating cookies non-stop. I decided that I needed to face my fears big and small and work through them.

Since *exercise* conjures up such negative emotions in some people, I prefer to call it *movement*. *Movement* is a much more user friendly word. "I can't exercise," my clients tell me. In reality, if you can sit in a chair and move your arms, you're exercising, because you're moving.

Let's dispense with the notion that you require a gym membership, workout clothes, a fitness tracker, a trainer, or lots of time in order to move. None of that is necessary. If you can function independently in your daily activities, you've got all that it takes to move your body toward better health.

The American Council on Exercise

I am certified by the American Council on Exercise (ACE) as a personal trainer. I maintain that certification so I can stay on top of the fast-changing world of exercise science. ACE is one of the leading organizations for fitness professional credentials. Founded in 1985, ACE is a nonprofit organization committed to America's health and wellbeing.

Over the past 30 years, they have become an established resource for health and fitness professionals and for the public, providing comprehensive, unbiased research and validating themselves as the country's trusted authority on health and fitness. Today, ACE is the largest nonprofit health and fitness certification, education, and training organization in the world, with more than 60,000 certified professionals who hold more than 67,000 ACE Certifications. With a long heritage in certification, education, training, and public outreach, they are among the most respected organizations in the industry and are a resource the public has come to trust for health and fitness education.

Today, ACE's mission is to get people moving. They have the philosophy that our nation needs a more prevention-centered way of caring for the health and wellness of its people, and safe, supervised physical activity must be a cornerstone.

ACE believes that well-qualified health and fitness professionals must become recognized as health providers and become authorized to provide prevention and wellness intervention services in the healthcare environment. It's about helping to keep people from getting sick in the first place, and helping those with chronic conditions to help themselves just a little bit more. I have a great deal of respect for this organization.

I Needed to Trust a Reliable Source

I had never worked with a trainer until I started my last weight loss attempt, and had zero medical background when I decided to become a personal trainer. At the age of 56, after a 27-year corporate career, and after losing 185 pounds, I began to study for the ACE exam. I had to learn about all of the muscles and joints in our bodies, all of their Latin names, and how each of them worked together to move us through life. It was brutal, but I did it, not so that I could train people for a living, but because I wanted to know exactly what I needed to do to maintain my new body. I wanted to know the truth, from an unbiased source, instead of falling for one of those late-night infomercials that wanted to sell me a new gadget every week that would reshape my butt, lift my boobs, and flatten my stomach.

I now know exactly how to reshape any body, and I can teach you how. But, again, as with the foods we eat, I can give you the knowledge, but I want to you learn how to apply it to your daily life in a way that makes sense *for you*. I want to teach you how to love moving your body toward better health.

"Why Is Exercise Important?"

In case you've never had the experience, let me tell you about the less obvious benefits of exercise – and it's not to burn off what you ate last night. After I realized that I wasn't going to die when I jumped on the elliptical machine, I was less skeptical and went back the next day and the next day and almost every day after that for a very long time. I soon found my little hole-in-the-wall gym to be a sanctuary. There I could zone out to my music and just walk on the treadmill. No one could reach me or drop in on my "me time." It was an escape. Go figure. It gave me time to be alone with my thoughts. That was a rarity for me. I began to look forward to my treadmill time and saved things that I had to think about until I could get on the treadmill. All of a sudden, I couldn't wait to get there. The more I did that the longer I was able to walk.

I Can Do This

I could feel the effects of movement immediately. Not in my dress size, but in my confidence level rising. I had slowly transitioned from someone who never exercised to someone who looked forward to it. All that really changed was how I thought about it. Instead of dreading it, I equated exercise time with "my time" and became very protective of it and proud of myself. I believed I could do it, when it used to seem impossible. *If I can do this, what else can I do?*

Exercise builds self-confidence and provides a sense of accomplishment.

Exercise Clears My Mind

I noticed my stress level coming down and learned that when I am feeling stressed or overwhelmed, if I can go for a quick brisk walk, I can refocus and be more productive. This technique has become part of my daily life. When I feel antsy or frustrated, I'll go for a quick walk, ride my bike, or go for a swim and, like magic, I'm refreshed.

As I became more conditioned, I was able to add inclines and to increase my speed. That's when I experienced *runner's high* for the first time. It was awesome and freaky at the same time. I was really working hard on the treadmill, sweating and breathing hard, and I could not speak a more than one word at a time, and then, all of a sudden, it was like my feet left the treadmill and I was soaring above it. Like when ET took flight across the night sky. The conversation in my head went like this: *Wow, this is awesome. This must be that runner's high.* As soon as I had that thought it was gone, and so was the feeling. But after that I wanted it again. *Is this how people get hooked on exercise?* I wondered. *This is the best new drug in the world. Who is this girl and what happened to the one who hated exercise?"*

That was how it started for me.

Exercise Builds Muscle

Of course exercise builds muscle, and that's the goal here. When you build muscle your body naturally burns more calories. Even when you're sleeping or sitting at your desk every day. Regular cardio exercise will lower your resting heart rate, which means that your heart doesn't have to work as hard to do its job of circulating your blood supply. And regular cardio exercise will burn calories. But don't think for a minute that you can lose weight and maintain it solely through exercising.

You Can't Outrun Your Fork

I remember reading about how this concept was proven when, under laboratory conditions, two men with equal body size and shape were tested for fifteen minutes to see who would total the most calories burned vs. eaten. The eater was served a whole pizza and the exerciser was hooked up to a specially equipped treadmill that accurately measures calorie burn, like a cardio stress test. *Ready, set, go.* I'm sure you can guess the outcome. The pizza guy put away six slices before he had to stop eating after consuming about 1800 calories, while the in-shape running guy burned less than 300 calories. Wow, look at how quickly we consume and how slowly we burn. Not fair! But those are the facts.

I can assure you that just about 100% of the clients I teach underestimate their calorie consumption and overestimate the value of their exercise. If this is you, you're not alone, and it isn't fair, but that's the truth. If you want to know exactly what you're burning, get a fitness tracker. It isn't necessary, but it makes a believer out of the skeptic once you see how hard you have to work to burn off that cute little cupcake someone left in the break room.

"How Should I Start My Exercise Plan?"

That's up to you. There is no right number of minutes on the treadmill or crunches to do. I know from experience that you must feel good about your exercise plan in order to stick with it. So many clients with good intentions come in with a plan to get to the gym five to six days a week for an hour each. They are the epitome of gung ho, but what we see instead is crash and burn. It is unrealistic to stick with a plan like that when currently you are doing zero exercise.

Make a Commitment to You

My advice to all my clients is to establish a minimum level of regular exercise that you can live with forever. Can you really see yourself getting to the gym that often for that long every week? If you have the slightest doubt, then don't set yourself up for failure. Start small; you can always bump it up. But when you put an impossible goal out there and fail to reach it the first time it takes you down the rabbit hole.

What's important to note is that by *regular exercise*, I don't mean going to the gym five times a week for an hour or training for a marathon. *Regular exercise* for you is whatever you choose to commit to. It could be walking for half an hour each morning, before work, or after dinner. This is your program to define and, as long as you stick with it, it will become a healthy habit.

You Can Do Anything for Five Minutes

Let's start by establishing your minimum commitment. Even if it's walking for five minutes a day. Or five minutes three times a week. Whatever seems entirely doable to you right now, put it on your calendar. That appointment with yourself is as important as an appointment with your most valuable client, your boss, or your doctor. Once you put it on your calendar it becomes non-negotiable, so think about this and then put it in stone.

I start each workout with a five-minute commitment, even to this day. When I reach the five minute mark, I decide if I want to do another five, and see how it goes. It's rare that I do less than forty minutes five times a week. That is more than enough to satisfy the minimum standard the government recommends to maintain good health, which is 150 minutes weekly of cardio exercise. This number sounded as impossible to achieve to me as climbing Mount Everest would. But 5 minutes a day? *That* I could do.

"How Do I know if I'm Doing Enough?"

I get this question a lot: "Why am I not losing weight, even though I walk for an hour five days a week?" That can be frustrating, and I wonder if I'd have enough persistence to stick with something if I weren't getting the results I expected. I have to admire these women who keep walking even though they see no changes.

There are two reasons why you may not see the expected results from your exercise: underestimating the calories burned by your exercise or underestimating the number of calories eaten in your diet.

First, you may be underestimating the calories burned by your exercise. If you can hold a conversation while you're walking, you need to turn it up a bit. Don't get me wrong, the fact that you're walking at all and for an hour is awesome. Your legs are strong and you are building muscle and you are burning more calories than you would be sitting on the couch.

If you're on a mission to lose weight and keep it off, try this: In the absence of a fitness tracker, notice how you are breathing when you exercise. How hard are you exerting yourself? On a scale from zero to ten what is your perceived exertion? If zero is *couch potato* and ten is *running for your life*, you need to be at about six to make a difference in your body. You'll know you're at a level six when you cannot sing while you're moving. At seven it becomes difficult to hold a conversation with the person on the next treadmill. Once you pass eight you can usually only spit out one syllable at a time. So, next time you go for a walk, check your rate of perceived exertion against the scale above and step it up to a six and stay in that zone for as long as you can.

There are many things you can to do continually challenge yourself as you become more conditioned, like adding inclines, ankle weights, or short bursts of running in between longer periods of walking. This technique is called *interval training.*

An example of interval training on the treadmill would look like this: Walk for five minutes at your normal treadmill pace, get your rate of perceived exertion up to level six, and then go all out for ten seconds. Run for your life. But only for ten seconds. Then bring it back down to level six again and walk for five minutes, then burst again. You can do this over and over. Try to lengthen the bursts of all-out running – or fast walking if your joints tell you not to run – and shorten the time in between bursts. I love this technique because it doesn't add any time to your workout but it is a more efficient way to get the benefits you're after.

The second reason you're not seeing a change in your body even though you're exercising regularly is because you are underestimating the number of calories in your diet. That's it. No mystery. You can't outrun your fork. So go back to your food diary, or start keeping one, and just watch what happens. I've never seen this effort fail to produce the desired results.

Be Realistic about Your Expectations

You can over exercise, so be careful when you plan your exercise program. Plan with the understanding that the habits you're forming will be with you for life. So many people expect too much from themselves and when they don't see immediate results from their exercise give it up in frustration or try to do more and more until they burn out or get injured. *Take your time and allow your new habit to find its rightful place in your life.*

Don't be fooled into thinking that exercise alone will be enough to make you lose weight successfully. If you're eating more than you're burning, the scale will continue to climb. The math always works.

Meet Roy

Roy is a letter-carrier who came to me to lose 50 pounds. He ate a relatively good diet and because he walked his 13-mile route each day he thought that was enough exercise to lose the weight. I pointed out that he had gained the weight in the past five years and he's been walking that route for 15 years, so it obviously wasn't just about the exercise. He never did any more exercise than walking his mail route. So, what had changed for Roy?

He'd gotten married. His wife loved to cook and prepared fabulous meals for him. Every night was a treat and, after five happy years of marriage, he was carrying another 50 pounds.

We changed some of his food habits, but it was when he started wearing ankle weights while he walked his route that things began to change. In about six months, the 50 pounds were gone!

"How Important is Strength Training?"

Most of my discussion here has centered on walking, but strength training – also known as resistance or weight training – is also important. I generally start my clients out with walking because they see the fastest results and that is very motivating.

Once you've gotten your cardio to a manageable place, I'd recommend strength training exercises twice a week. This can be as simple as doing a few squats as you brush your teeth in the morning and at night. It doesn't matter what time of day you do it, so do it when you feel it best fits into your daily routine. Again, it requires nothing fancy in terms of gear or gadgets. Your own body weight is all you need.

The reason to incorporate strength training sessions into your routine once or twice a week is because this is the type of exercise helps sculpt and tone your body. As you build muscle and lose fat, the muscle tone you develop begins to show in your shape as muscle definition. You will see that your arms look more cut and there's definition in your abs.

In addition, every pound of muscle you build is burning more calories for you even while you're at rest. This is why some women can eat more food or more calories and still maintain their shape. Their bodies are naturally burning more calories per hour than the next woman. This is also why, pound for pound, men can eat so much more than women and also lose weight so quickly. It isn't fair, but it's true. Their body composition is naturally skewed toward more muscle than fat, and women are the complete opposite.

You need to know that you cannot lose weight only in your arms or your belly. It doesn't work like that. No amount of sit ups will flatten your abs if you are not losing fat all over your body. Don't fall for that line of sales hype. Stay away from those late night infomercials that try to sell you another useless piece of equipment. It will end up under your bed or as a clothing rack and will be a constant reminder of another failed attempt. It's not helpful, so don't waste your time or money.

Hire a Trainer

I'm all for hiring a trainer if you can afford it. It makes the commitment to move even harder to break when you know there is someone waiting for you to show up for your workout. A trainer will push you and, most importantly, make sure you are exercising in a safe and effective way.

There are a number of ways you can begin a relationship with a trainer. Establishing a good client-trainer relationship can be instrumental in helping you stick with your program. Always look for your potential trainer though a reputable source.

Although I do not train clients, I recommend trainers who maintain current American Council on Exercise Personal Trainer credentials. Go to www.acefitness.org and use their find a trainer feature to see trainers in your area. Ask questions, be honest about your concerns and give yourself time to try it out for a few weeks before you make a decision to stick with this person or to find someone else.

Your fist session with an ACE professional will involve assessments and information-gathering. A good trainer needs to know a lot about you before they start working on building your program. Establishing a good rapport is critical, so don't settle for someone you don't relate to. Keep looking until you find a good match.

Expect your trainer to push you a little past where you might go on your own as you work together and as you get stronger, but never push you to the point of injury. You should be able to trust that your trainer will always be looking out for your safety first.

Ideally, you'll be able to meet with them twice a week for resistance training. By adding resistance training to your minimum cardio commitment you will have created an effective, realistic exercise program that you can maintain for a lifetime.

A Tale of Two Clients

I've got two clients, Maria and Joan, who are both about 60 years old, around 5'2", and weigh about 135 pounds, which gives them a "normal" body mass index (BMI) of about 24.3. "Normal" is a term I object to, but these are the standards established by the World Health Organization. A person whose BMI is between 18.5 and 24.9 is in the "normal" range. Above 25 is considered "overweight,", and a BMI over 30 is classified as "obese."

Your BMI is calculated using only two numbers: your height and your weight. Unless and until we can figure out how to grow a few inches taller at this point in life, the only way to get a better BMI is to drop some pounds.

Maria and Joan have two very different lifestyles, and it shows in their shapes. They both lost about 40 pounds by working with me over the course of a year. What is so remarkable about these two women is how different their bodies look. They both would be considered at a "good weight" by our societal norms, and this is further supported by the normal BMI reading.

Maria and Joan both have sedentary jobs where they sit at a desk most days. But the similarities end there. Joan walks the ten blocks from her train stop to her office and back again most days. That amounts to one mile a day five days a week. Joan also loves to dance and will go out at least two nights a month dancing with her husband. She loves to stay active on the weekends, so she is always either playing a round of golf (with no golf cart) or going biking or hiking in the park. And she has a trainer she sees twice a week. She looks toned and athletic and years younger than her chronological age.

What's so funny about Joan is that if you ask her what kind of exercise she does to stay in such great shape, she only mentions the two times a week with her trainer. The other things she does are just part of her life. She does these things because she likes to.

Maria, on the other hand, admits that she hates to exercise. She'd rather go to a movie with her hubby after a dinner out on the weekends or backgammon with the girls once a week. She wouldn't consider hiring a trainer, which seems like a luxury, something a movie star would do.

Maria and Joan are both able to successfully maintain their weight loss by eating a healthy, clean diet. So why does Joan wear a size four to six and Maria a size ten? It's because Joan's weight is more muscle than fat. Since fat takes up more room in your clothes, Maria needs a bigger size and her overall appearance is soft and round, while Joan's is toned and trim. Both are healthy and don't need to change a thing as long as they are satisfied with what they see in the mirror. The difference in their shapes is due to the ratio of fat-to-lean in their bodies.

What to Eat before and After Exercise

In order to get the most from your workout, plan to have a small snack about half an hour before beginning. This snack should fit within your daily calorie allowance and consist of a food that is relatively high in complex carbs, to maximize your blood glucose availability, and low in fat and fiber to minimize gastrointestinal distress. A small granola-type bar or a whole wheat mini-bagel are my two favorite choices. A small amount of protein is tolerated well by some, so try it and see for yourself.

About 30 minutes after your workout, the best meals include carbs and proteins. The carbs will replace the energy used in your work out and the protein will help repair your muscles. But be careful – not all carbs are created equal, and you want to pick something like raisins for the quick-release of sugar.

After all is said and done, increasing your daily activity while moderately reducing your total daily calorie consumption is still the best way to move the scale down and keep it there.

To Do

Calendar your exercise to take place at a time of day that suits you. As you try to figure out what time is best, move it around to different hours and days in the week to see if you prefer a particular time or day over another. We are all different, so don't worry about what works for your friend or sister; just figure out when you can realistically fit it in. Establish your minimum exercise commitment and add that to your calendar or food diary.

Consider hiring a trainer.

IIIIIIIIIIIIIIIIIIIIIIIIIIIIII

Chapter 8
"Stressed?"

I prefer to handle stress naturally, without drugs or alcohol, and so I want to give you some ways that have worked for me and my clients. I suggest you give each a try for about four days to see for yourself whether that idea works. Or perhaps you'll come up with some new method that works even better for you.

The Power of Your Mind

Let me first demonstrate the power of your mind to change your body. Imagine that I had a really big, juicy lemon on my cutting board and I sliced into it with a big chef's knife. I raise half the lemon to my mouth and take a big bite out of it as the juice flows out and dribbles down my arm.

Eeeew.

Did you feel it? Did you feel the tingling in your jaw, did you start to salivate? Did you pucker or cringe? That was a physical reaction in your body that was created only by the thought you had about the words on this page. Nothing else. We're not in the same room and you couldn't see me cut the lemon or smell the lemon oils in the air, yet your thoughts about my words caused a physical reaction in you.

Can you see how what you think about things has a tremendous effect on your body?

Instead of "managing stress" I'd rather you not create it in the first place. Many people think stress happens *to* them, but I think we choose to be stressed. I know it may seem odd to think about stress this way. Do you know some people who never seem to lose their cool, no matter what happens? And then there are others who seem to have a black cloud following them everywhere and run around constantly with their hair on fire? There's a reason for that. Once you understand that you feel stressed when you *chose* to think about things in a way that is upsetting, you realize that you can *choose* to think about the same thing in a way that is more settling, pleasing, and even fun.

Meet Jane

Jane was a client who came to me to lose 50 pounds. She was a brilliant woman with her PhD in nursing and had just retired from being a professor of nursing. Jane was completely miserable about the prospect of spending long weekends at her new husband's beach house in the coming season. She didn't swim, snorkel, or water ski, because of her bad knees, but all his friends were avid participants in all of those water sports.

She felt she didn't fit in. She couldn't imagine how she could enjoy the time there with "Nothing to do, while everyone else has a good time." But, to be a sport, she'd agreed to go. She couldn't sleep after making that decision. She was stress-eating and barking at her husband. Why? She wasn't even at the beach house yet and she was anticipating how miserable she was going to be. She was choosing to be stressed at that moment. The thought of going there was so distasteful to her that she created the upset she was feeling.

I asked Jane to close her eyes and describe how it felt in her body when she pictured herself alone at the beach house waiting for everyone to come back after their day on the water. "Sick to my stomach" is how she described it. We were in my office in the city on a bright, sunny autumn afternoon and she was sick to her stomach over something that hadn't happened yet. She was choosing to feel that way at that moment and it affected her physically with an actual upset stomach.

I asked her, "How would you like to feel about those long beach house weekends? Can you imagine a scenario where you could have a good time doing things you love while everyone else was boating?"

"I guess so" was her reply.

So I asked, "How does your stomach feel now?"

"Not so bad."

We didn't find answers for Jane's choice of activities while she's at the beach house that session, but what she learned was that she could choose the thought to create a better feeling and, when she did, she would be a lot less stressed and able to make better choices.

Challenge Your Beliefs

The idea that we can challenge our own beliefs comes as news to people, so you may to object to this, but the truth is the stress we feel comes from our beliefs, from our thoughts. The things we hold on to as truths – no matter where we picked them up – form the basis against which we judge our successes or failures, our self-worth, and our level of acceptance.

Think about where your stress comes from and start asking yourself important questions. What are you feeling on a daily basis? Are these feelings serving you? How would you like to feel?

Be Grateful

Thinking about your blessings and the things you are grateful for can help to reduce stress. This may be difficult in the beginning, so try to find something you are truly thankful for. Start by making a list of those things.

I like to keep a gratitude journal and I often refer to it when I felt down or alone. It helps to remind me that I have much to be grateful for.

My gratitude journal started with: *I am happy to be alive.* I couldn't come up with much more in the early days of my weight loss! I was so numb to feeling anything that I couldn't see that I had a lot of love and support and I had (and still have) a terrific husband. I had much more than I realized. Every now and then, when I was having a bad day, I'd go to my journal and re-read the things I'd already written to remind myself that I was, indeed, very fortunate.

Try a Massage

We now have scientific proof of the benefits of massage – benefits ranging from treating chronic diseases and injuries to alleviating the growing tensions of our modern lifestyles. Having a massage does more than just relax your body and mind. There are specific physiological and psychological changes that occur during a massage, even more so when massage is utilized as a preventative, frequent therapy and not merely luxury.

Massage not only feels good, but it can cure what ails you. Evidence is showing that the more massage you allow yourself, the better you'll feel. The most recent studies have shown that the same pleasure-sensing areas of your brain that are satisfied by foods can also be satisfied by touch.

Massage as a healing tool has been around for thousands of years in many cultures. Touching is a natural human reaction to pain and stress, and for conveying compassion and support. Think of the last time you bumped your head or had a sore calf. What did you do? Rubbed it, right? The same was true for our earliest ancestors. Healers throughout time and throughout the world have instinctually and independently developed a wide range of therapeutic techniques using touch. Many are still in use today, and for good reason.

It is estimated that 80% to 90% of disease is stress-related. Massage can help reduce that percentage by providing much-needed relaxation.

The physical changes massage brings to your body can have a positive effect in many areas of your life. Besides increasing relaxation and helping to decrease anxiety, massage lowers blood pressure, increases circulation, improves recovery from injury, helps improves sleeping, and can increase concentration. It reduces fatigue and provides more energy for handling stressful situations.

Acupuncture

Acupuncture – a treatment that uses thin needles on the body's energy meridians – helps to prevent illness by improving the overall functioning of the body's immune and organ systems. It's helpful for treating existing illnesses and injuries, preventing illness and the recurrence of illness, and improving overall health.

Acupuncture originated in Asia over 3,000 years ago and is part of the holistic system of healing known as Traditional Chinese Medicine. The classical Chinese explanation for why acupuncture works is that energy (Qi) flows in channels (meridians) throughout the body and over its surfaces. These channels are rivers of energy. The Chinese have identified 12 meridians in the human body, which provides a basic energy map for all people. The meridians are often compared to a series of interconnected highways. Each of the major organs in the body is associated with its own meridian. Through the network of meridians, the internal organs are connected to certain areas and parts of the body, including the muscles, bones, joints, and other organs.

The Chinese believe that health is a manifestation of balance, both within the body itself and between the body and the external environment. When the body is internally balanced and in harmony with the external environment, Qi flows smoothly through the meridians to nourish the organs and tissues. If an obstruction occurs in one of the meridians, the Qi is disrupted and cannot flow properly. When the Qi cannot flow smoothly or is forced to flow in the opposite direction, the body's innate balance is disrupted and illness results.

Acupuncture points are the specific points on the meridians where the Qi is both concentrated and accessible. Acupuncture engages the Qi by inserting thin needles at these specific points, the goal being to restore the proper flow of Qi. As the body regains its natural balance, well-being returns.

To the human body, acupuncture needles are a physical stimulus. When the body detects this change, it produces a response. Although acupuncture is not yet fully understood by Western science, with modern technology scientists can now actually begin to "see" the body's response to acupuncture. For example, using an MRI, researchers have shown that when a needle is inserted at specific acupuncture points on the body, corresponding changes occur in the brain.

Acupuncture is most well-known for its ability to relieve pain, so the majority of research thus far has been done in that area. Acupuncture points are now believed to stimulate the central nervous system (the brain and spinal cord) to release pain-relieving chemicals into the muscles, spinal cord, and brain. Acupuncture may also stimulate other chemicals to be released by the brain, including hormones that influence the self-regulating system of the body.

Oriental medicine has been around for thousands of years and has provided us with a unique and holistic approach to help prevent and treat disease. Western science and Traditional Chinese Medicine ultimately rely on the body's natural healing ability to maintain health and protect against disease. Both have the same goal of helping a person stay healthy. Western science tends to use drugs and surgery as preferences. Acupuncturists tend to use gentle needling and herbs. A combination of both systems creates an ideal environment of health and healing.

Acupuncture, for me, was a big departure from the traditional Western medical approach I had been using my entire life. In the skilled hands of Dr. Joseph D'Antona, DOAM, acupuncture was instrumental in helping me reduce stress in my life and the toll it was taking on my body. The decision to try it was part of my plan to try something different to see if it would help and if I could envision making it part of my new, healthy lifestyle.

I had my first acupuncture treatment in July of 2008, when I weighed over 320 pounds. It was initially a bit scary and intimidating for someone who was in the habit of passing out when I had my blood drawn. But I was quickly put at ease after seeing how flexible the needles were and how kind and caring my doctor was. He listened to me. That may not seem like a big deal, but when I'd presented my 300-plus-pound self to most every medical practitioner in the past, I'd felt that all they saw was my size, and they never spoke to the person hiding inside. For the first time in my life, I felt valued and respected as a complete human being.

As I left Dr. D'Antona's office after my first treatment, I felt like I floated above the ground. Never in my life had I experienced such deep relaxation. It was a feeling of freedom that was both blissful and fleeting – and something I had to have more of.

I have grown to trust Dr. D'Antona to treat me wherever the stress in my body has taken up residence that week, to help me quickly recover from two joint replacements and several skin removal surgeries that followed my weight loss. I am devoted to receiving weekly acupuncture treatments. This is an important element of my self-care regimen, so it's a non-negotiable appointment on my calendar. I hope that you will seek out this type care and are as fortunate as I was to find a skilled local practitioner in your community.

To Do

Start a gratitude journal. A notebook is fine for some, while others prefer the digital way. Whichever you decide, make sure your journal is never far from you. Write in it every day. Date the page and write down one thing you are grateful for each day. Promise yourself you'll do this every day.

Treat yourself to a weekly massage. Find a massage therapist you are comfortable with and put it on your calendar to have a massage once a week, if possible, but at a minimum twice monthly.

Investigate the availability of acupuncture. Check to see what's available in your area. Some health plans are now covering acupuncture and, if you are so fortunate, use this benefit to your advantage.

Chapter 9

Hydration

The role water plays in the body is critical, yet most of my clients come to me dehydrated. They all know the old adage to drink eight glasses of water a day, but is that right for you? And how much is "a glass," anyway? It depends who's pouring, right?

Are You Dehydrated?

A state of dehydration will show up as fatigue, muscle cramps, hunger, lack of focus, irritability, and headaches, to name a few symptoms. Does this sound like you at 4:00 pm? Then take a drink of water. In order to be properly hydrated, you need to drink the equivalent of half your body weight in ounces of water. So if you weigh 200 pounds, you need 100 ounces of water a day. How close are you coming to that target?

Meet Hallie

If you find you're like my client Hallie, you have lots of catching up to do. Hallie is a smart businesswoman who has had a difficult time losing weight and now weighs 330 pounds. We are working on getting her food choices and portions under control, but her hydration is something that is keeping her from being successful. How can that be?

Based on her weight, she needs to be drinking 165 ounces of water daily – that's more than a gallon – and she drinks zero water! How is that even possible? She drinks coffee, wine, and diet soda. That's it. The thought of drinking water brings up reasons why she can't: "I'll have to pee all day and I take the train, so I don't have time to pee, and I can't carry that much water around all day." She went on and on with all the reasons it would be impossible for her to drink that much water.

Just a Little Better Than Yesterday

I get it. Drinking a lot when you haven't been drinking any sounds like a drastic change. But here's an idea: Why not try challenging yourself to add just one 16-ounce bottle of water per day this week. Can you do that? Even if it takes all day to drink it, that will be an improvement over what you did last week. That's all it really takes – just doing a little bit more than you did yesterday, until you reach your target.

Hallie agreed to my water challenge, and we made it interesting by making a deal. If she drank one 16-ounce bottle of water each day for a week, she would buy herself an expensive new lipstick. If she didn't reach her goal, she would buy it anyway, but give it to a friend as a gift. This worked like a charm in week one, so we pushed the envelope and made the goal two bottles of water each day for the next week. And each time she met her challenge we increased the reward and the penalty.

We got pretty creative with rewards. They were always self-indulgent body pampering or experiences, never dinner out or a bottle of wine. We pushed and pushed for weeks, until she got there. She felt confident that she would get there, because we took it slowly. Hallie began to notice that her headaches were not as frequent or severe, her leg cramps were gone, and she had more energy throughout the day.

Hallie became an advocate of drinking water, especially when I taught her how to make fruit infused waters of all kinds. And, guess what? Without the fatigue, she was better able to move her body, and when the headaches cleared up and gave her peace from the pain that ignited the desire to treat herself better. The change in her was remarkable and so simple: Drink water.

Water Retention

There's another benefit of being well hydrated that often goes unnoticed and can easily derail the most dedicated of us. When we don't get adequate water our brilliant body thinks we're dying of thirst and goes into protection mode. It holds onto the water we've currently got on hand and we bloat – we retain water. I know this is totally counterintuitive, but that amazing body of yours is designed to protect you and it's only doing its job. You know those days when your rings are stuck or your ankles are swollen. Start drinking water and the issue will likely resolve.

When you're in a state of retaining water, the scale goes up a few pounds. It doesn't matter if you've been eating according to your food plan and exercising too. If you're retaining even a quart of water the scale will show two more pounds than yesterday. Water weighs about eight pounds per gallon. This can really cause a lot of confusion when you're expecting the scale to go down and instead it goes up.

Combine a lack of water with eating salty foods and *wham*, instant temporary facelift. Truly, your face will puff up and all those annoying lines will disappear for a short time. But don't be tempted to try this before your cousin's wedding; if you're anything like me, you'll end up with puffy bags under your eyes – not pretty.

How to Make Infused Water

Did you ever go to a spa and see all those pretty water containers with fresh fruits and herbs in them? They look so thirst-quenching, and they taste even better. Making water flavored with fruits and vegetables – infused water – is easy.

There are many reasons why infused water is beneficial as a beverage:

- It is easy to make.
- It is virtually calorie-free.
- There is no diet soda aftertaste.
- It is inexpensive.
- It is a great way to use up extra produce items or to take advantage of store sales.

Four Steps to Making Infused Water

1. Decide which flavors you want to use. The sky's the limit! Choose cucumber, tomato, mint, berries, melons, or citrus fruits, for example. But avoid items like apples or pears, which turn brown. It is best to slice your items thinly.

2. Make your mix by pouring warm water into a pitcher. Add the flavor items. Generally speaking, the ratio is about one cup of fruits or vegetables to about two quarts of warm water. Mix the water and other ingredients together.

3. Cover and put in the refrigerator. Allow to sit for about 2-3 hours or overnight. Shelf life will vary depending on what ingredients you use, but generally you can keep your infused water for a couple of days. If you remove the ingredients after a day or two it might last a little longer.

4. Pour over ice and enjoy! If you want to take your infused water with you on the go, simply store it in an insulated cup with some ice.

Flavor Ideas

- Cucumber with lime
- Lemon and/or orange
- Mixed berries and mint
- Grapefruit
- Watermelon
- Lemon and raspberry
- Cucumber and green tea

To Do

Track your water consumption for four days. How much water do you drink, on average? This is your baseline and the place from which we'll start to bring your water consumption up to the appropriate level. Wherever you start, if you're not already drinking the right amount for you, we can always improve things a bit. So, if you're only drinking two glasses of water a day and now realize you need ten, please don't think you have to get there overnight. Just add one glass per day until that new level seems normal, then add one more glass per day. Eventually you'll get there.

Ask for help. You don't have to do any of this alone when I'm happy to help you figure it out. Just drop me an email at Debbie@debbielazinsky.com.

||||||||||||||||||||||||||||||||

Chapter 10

Appreciate the Process

O nce I realized that dieting wasn't the answer and that I'd
always need to pay attention to what I was eating, a cold
chill ran through my body. It was as if I had been given
a life sentence. But it was at that same moment when I told myself
that if this is what it's going to take to live a full, healthy life, then
I'd better learn to appreciate the *process* instead of only focusing on
the end goal. Otherwise, I'd always be chasing a long-term goal. I
knew enough about myself to know that I needed to see continuous
progress or I'd lose interest. I would have to use short-term goals on
my way to the final goal, which, for me, was not a number on the
scale. I just wanted to live to see 60.

This Is Not a Diet – It's How I Eat Now

This shift – from "on a diet" to "this is how I eat now" – was a major mind shift for me. It was a relief to know that there was no deadline or urgency any longer. It wasn't about hanging on until I got to the finish line. This was my life *now*, and why would I want to wish it away? I was already 56 years old, so I wasn't going to wish away any of my remaining days.

"This is how I eat now, this is not a diet."

That is when I really settled into a healthy routine. I had to face the fact that there were things I needed to do every day and every week to take care of myself. They are as vitally important to my health as brushing my teeth every day. I needed to eat well, get enough sleep, drink enough water, get some form of movement into my day, and effectively deal with stressful situations.

Why hadn't I ever learned this on my own before? I didn't know, but I did know that no one had ever taught me the importance of self-care. It was as if I was supposed to know it instinctively or absorb it from the environment. But I hadn't, and it had never occurred to me that I needed to care for my body in this way. As I gained more awareness, I kept learning more and was able to teach myself how to better care for myself.

Sticking with the Plan Was My Goal

I began to find accomplishment in sticking with my plan and knowing I was taking the best care of myself that I possibly could. I felt an unfamiliar sense of calm and control. Anytime I'd find myself distracted from my new healthy habits, I'd remind myself to just stick with the process.

I had a well-considered plan in place, and it was my responsibility to trust the plan and find at least a tiny victory in each day. Yes, the end goal was inevitable if I stuck with the plan. That was never in doubt.

It was my belief in the process – more than my belief in me – that sustained my motivation on many days.

Realistic Goal-Setting

Anyone who holds a college degree or executive position knows the importance of applying realistic goal-setting to your work. It's a skill we use daily in our business lives, yet we may not carry it over and put it to use in our personal lives. But goal-setting is a transferrable skill. And one you're probably already good at. So let's put it to use.

Be SMART

Set realistic, SMART goals. SMART is an acronym for goals that are specific, measurable, attainable, relevant, and time-bound. An example of a SMART goal is: "I will walk for one mile on five days this week." This is not a SMART goal: "I'm going to start exercising this week." It's just too vague and non-specific. It's more like wishful thinking. I find that if I write down my SMART goals, they are more real and attainable.

Set Yourself on Autopilot

Once walking a mile a day on most days a week becomes an ingrained habit, like brushing your teeth, you will no longer feel that it is an imposition or something you have to put too much mental energy into. Really, it just becomes part of what you do. There's no question about whether you'll do it every day. You don't spend any time complaining about how much you hate it or how long it takes. You just do it. Maybe Nike was on to something.

When you set out on this journey to get healthy and then realize just how many things in your life need to change, it can be overwhelming to think about it in totality. This is where the aspect of goal-setting is critically important.

When I realized I had to lose almost 200 pounds, I could not imagine where or how to start, so I decided to do just one thing differently until that became a habit, and then I would start another new habit, and then another one.

"How Can I Create New Habits?"

One method for creating new habits that worked well for me was to attach a new desired behavior to one that was already a habit. For example, brushing my teeth was something I did without fail in the morning and before bed. I decided that when I was brushing my teeth I would do ten squats. I wasn't doing *any* exercise at the time, so 20 squats a day was a big jump. What If I could only do five? That was okay, because as long as I did some, I'd eventually work up to ten. That's when I committed to my squat routine. I still do it. But now I do 20 in the morning and 20 in the evening. I almost have a hard time brushing my teeth and not doing them, because my brain has connected the two.

I began to create a chain of good habits all connected to brushing my teeth in the morning and in the evening. I now have a morning routine that includes walking on my treadmill, eating a great breakfast, doing my squats, setting my intentions for the day, drinking a big glass of water, and writing in my journal. It happens like clockwork. I struggle to break out of this routine when I have to catch an early flight or need to get to an early doctor appointment. It's really funny how these habits have taken over.

My evening routine has morphed into my sleep ritual. It starts with brushing my teeth right after dinner. That's the signal that we are done eating for the day. I'm not going to be brushing my teeth again after a late snack. Then I turn off my phone and computer and I read, stretch, take a lavender bath (if I have time), and have a cup of hot water with lemon. These habits have become part of me, too. This is what I do to take care of myself, and it's not a chore that I wish would end, and I don't hope for the day when I won't have to do them anymore.

I take comfort in my routines now and feel that I deserve this bit of pampering so that I can be 100% of who I am supposed to be for my husband, my friends, and my clients. I owe it to the people who are counting on me to take good care of myself. The good health, crazy amount of energy, and positive outlook I enjoy are my rewards for developing new healthy habits. And, by the way, when you spend time practicing your new habits, they tend to crowd out the ones that may have been working against you in the past.

Rewards System

Many of my clients respond well to a reward system. I used non-food rewards as my incentive in the early days. If I stuck with the process, if I met my SMART goal, I'd reward myself accordingly. If you find this motivating, then draw up a contract with yourself that goes something like this: *I am going to walk for one mile each day for five days this week. If I do, I will treat myself to a manicure and pedicure at the new salon in town.* Then do it. Treat yourself to something you wouldn't normally indulge in. Make it fun and interesting by telling a trusted friend what you're up to. I kept pushing the envelope with my goals and rewards.

I rewarded myself for every ten pounds I lost, which was about once a month. I'd start the month by setting my sights on the reward and then getting to work. I would stick with my plan and then, at the end of the month, I'd get on the scale and see if the work I had done was enough to collect my reward. If I didn't make my goal, I wouldn't collect. I'm happy to report that I hit my goal every time. In the beginning, I had big doubts, but along the way I began to believe in myself as much as I believed in my plan. I lost ten pounds a month, every month, for 18 consecutive months.

At 50 pounds down, I decided to accept an opportunity to appear on a national TV show. That was a big deal for someone who hid from the camera and would rather have an organ removed than speak in public (so much so that I once scheduled my gall bladder surgery on the same day I was supposed to do a big presentation at work. My former boss is just finding this out if he's reading this book. I'm sorry, Dave.) I felt this was a well-deserved reward. I was really proud of the 50 pounds I'd lost, and my confidence level was soaring at the time. If I ever was going to conquer my fears of public speaking and being photographed, that seemed like the best opportunity. So I did it!

The pounds kept melting away, and I kept reaching for bigger, more challenging, even scary, experiences to reward myself with. At 100 pounds down, I went skydiving (that's another story). The biggest reward was presented after I had lost it all, when *People* magazine picked me for their "Half My Size" issue. Wow! I was evolving into the person I was supposed to be, day by day, step by step, pound by pound.

The fog cleared, my priorities became focused, and life got so much simpler in some respects and so much richer in others. Once I had settled into my new habits, I was finally at peace with my body. I knew I was going to live.

Chapter 11

"Are You an Emotional Eater?"

There were so many emotions that drove my weight gain. I overate when I was in pain and uncomfortable in some way. I overate to numb my pain and seek pleasure. I felt like I had no way to stop myself and often ate until I was bursting and the food didn't even taste good any more. It was no longer giving me pleasure, yet I felt like I didn't know how to stop. I was like an addict seeking the "high" of pleasure.

In the same way we seek pleasure, we also try to avoid pain. We do this by distracting ourselves from uncomfortable feelings by overeating food we don't need or even want, or by overdrinking, over-shopping, or overworking. These can be very effective distractions, because as long as we are focused on the food or the diversionary "drug of choice" – how good it tastes or feels – we don't have to experience the discomfort of whatever emotion we might be feeling. We continuously use this technique to avoid pain and discomfort and, over time, it becomes cemented in our unconscious as a habit that may seem impossible to break.

It finally occurred to me that I could never fill a hole in my heart with food. Nothing in the world could ever taste good enough to make me happy for any longer than the time the taste lingered in my mouth. This revelation came with sadness at first, because I realized that I was chasing an imaginary prize. Food could never really make me feel the happiness I was seeking. Then I felt lost. If food wasn't the answer to total bliss, then what was?

It would take years to find out that I held the solution all along, just like Dorothy in *The Wizard of Oz*.

The Good News and the Bad News

The good news is that we *learned* to eat emotionally – we were not born with the natural instinct to use food for pleasure or to soothe pain. And so, if we learned this habit we can learn a better habit. Typically, clients think emotional eating means you break up with your boyfriend and you jump into a bathtub of Ben & Jerry's, but it's much more subtle than that. You could be slightly bored and grab for a handful of almonds, like Tom did, or maybe you've just given a big presentation at work and you feel you deserve to go out and celebrate. This is emotional eating and can be pre-empted once you recognize the signs and understand that your physical feelings of hunger are coming from the thought you are having.

There are several tools I'll teach you to help you recognize the difference between physical hunger and emotional hunger. I promise you that those two things can feel exactly the same, which is why this can be difficult to sort out. Let me first explain how we lost touch with our natural ability to tell the difference between the two.

We are born with a natural instinct to eat when we are physically hungry and stop eating when our physical hunger is satisfied. Notice that I did not say "when we are full." For some reason, we as a society have decided that children need to eat on their parents' schedule and eat the volume that we as parents think they should eat. This usually has little to do with getting the baby the nutrition needed and more about an arbitrary schedule that's forced upon them.

Did you ever try to give a baby a bottle when they aren't hungry? They try to avoid you by turning their head from side to side. They want nothing to do with it and this can frustrate a new mom who thinks she must feed her child now, or else. Stress builds in the mom and is transferred to the child immediately. By the same token, try taking a bottle away from a hungry baby and they clamp down on the nipple and won't let go.

At that point in your life, you were in touch with your internal hunger and satisfaction cues. That was pure physical hunger and satisfaction communication from baby to mother, with no chance the child is asking for food because she had a bad day or was bored.

When adults start to impose a schedule on a child for reasons of convenience or due to our own beliefs about food, we plant the seeds of emotional eating.

Meet Lisa

Lisa can remember playing in her backyard, which was really two lots side by side, since her grandparents lived next door. There were woods thick with blueberry bushes, lady slippers, and snapping turtles. She and her brother would set out on great adventures that seemed like they were really hiking through woods and living off the land. In fact, the two lots combined were only one fenced in acre of land, but to a six-year-old and a four-year-old it might as well have been a national park.

They'd set out after breakfast with their PB and J's and climb the trees, eat blueberries, and have the best time digging holes until they hit the water table and the hole would start to fill. They'd find a turtle to swim in the hole. They'd be out there for hours having the best time and then they'd hear a voice in the distance. "Lisa, Jimmy, where are you? Hurry up. Dinner is on the table."

They'd reluctantly give up on their nature hike and sit down to dinner, already stuffed on blueberries and *so* not into whatever Mom had cooked. The dinner table became a battle of wills. "Finish everything on your plate or you'll eat it for breakfast." *Yikes, those lima beans were pretty awful already, so how horrible would they be on my plate instead of my usual Fruit Loops for breakfast*, Lisa thought. So she would swallow them whole, with a big gulp of soda to make them disappear. Not fun, and probably the foundation for her emotional eating habits.

Can you see how this emotional manipulation caused Lisa to preempt her hunger/satisfaction signal and mingled it with the feelings of guilt or frustration? Many of my clients had similar pressures applied to them about food and eating. I know I did.

I Never Put People on a Diet

Many of my clients are confused when, instead of putting them on a diet and taking their favorite foods off the table, I work to help them think differently about how they manage their food in stressful or social situations. They soon realize that when they choose another way of dealing with pain and find pleasure in non-food experiences, emotional overeating decreases gradually and naturally. There is no need to tell them what to eat or how much. They naturally only eat enough to satisfy their physical hunger, and the excess weight melts away. This is so much more peaceful than trying to fight off your favorite foods with willpower. We all know that never works.

The Hunger Scale

I'm a big advocate of food journaling, but there are times when that's just not practical; or you've learned how to manage your choices and portions and you want to move away from your food diary. For those times, the Hunger Scale is a good tool.

Think of your hunger on a scale from minus ten to plus ten. In the middle is zero. At zero you're neither hungry nor full; you are satisfied, focused, and energetic. Plus one is somewhat satisfied, and plus two is where I encourage you to stop eating. A few bites after plus two you will begin to feel the food in your belly, and if you continue after that you will be moving into the overly fed zones of plus four and up.

When you assess your hunger at a minus two or three, I encourage having a small meal of about 150 to 300 calories, depending on your needs. But here's the trick: As you eat, do so slowly and notice when you are no longer in the minus two zone. A few more bites and you're at minus one, and then soon you're at zero, and that's when I want you to stop eating – just as soon as you no longer feel the hunger you felt before you started eating. You won't be "full," and you may not even feel satisfied, but you will feel different in about 15 minutes, because it can take that long for the satisfaction to register. You will be amazed at how little food you really need to be satisfied.

By consistently using the new tools you're learning, they will soon become part of your new healthy habits lifestyle. Notice when you're feeling the familiar twinge of discomfort that usually signals you to eat and use it instead as a warning sign that maybe you're stressed or bored and see if you can find another remedy. And, when you do eat, be mindful of each bite and stop when you get to zero or plus one, at the most, on the Hunger Scale.

Try this for four days and see if you can start to get back in touch with your natural hunger cues. When you feel the twinge of hunger, check in with your food journal to see how much and when you last ate. If there is no physical reason why your body should need food, then this is emotional hunger. Watch how often this comes up for you and how many different emotions can trigger this desire to eat.

I Can Manage My Feelings

You are creating your emotional hunger. This was great news to me. If I created it, then I could control it. OMG, this was big. Try it yourself and see how may decisions about food you make each day based on reasons other than nutrition. That's all emotional eating.

When you know you're dealing with an emotional need to eat, it will take some practice to grab hold of the feeling and work through it. I'm realistic enough to realize that there will be times when I will be tempted to eat emotionally. When the decision to eat emotionally pops us, as a creature of habit we may feel powerless against the pull of these old, deeply imbedded habits.

Arm Yourself

I wanted to be prepared for the next time my emotional hunger was sniffing around for satisfaction. One way that worked well for me was to keep a supply of air-pop popcorn. That was a food that looked really big in the bowl and smelled really good. It was crunchy and salty and I could keep eating and eating it. It was a big help, because at least the popcorn wasn't as fattening as the ice cream or peanut butter cups.

Once I started to conquer the habit of eating emotionally, I decided that I wanted to manage my emotions differently. That's when I really began substituting non-food experiences for emotional eating.

Use Your Senses

I found that indulging my other senses, besides taste, was similarly satisfying, and would keep me on my weight-loss track. If I found myself bored and drawn to the kitchen, I'd substitute another activity that was as satisfying as cooking was to me. I love to cook and would lose myself in creating a new recipe or technique. I loved the creative process of combining different tastes, and I loved the smell of delicious food, I also loved sharing food with my friends and family. I was drawn to aromatherapy as a substitute. It checked so many boxes for me. I found myself lost in the creative process, creating new recipes for lotions, soaps, scrubs, and oils. I loved giving them as gifts and my friends loved receiving them, too.

What Is Your Passion?

What do you lose track of time doing? How about doing that instead of eating when you feel drawn to emotional eating? Is there some way you can indulge your emotional need in a way that does not involve food?

In the beginning of my weight loss program, I ask my clients to make a list of non-food-related indulgences – things, experiences, and activities that soothe the emotion that needs attention, but will not add excess pounds to the body. It's even better if you *can't* eat while doing them. Here are some of these activities that are on my list:

- Take a shower or bubble bath.
- Go for a swim.
- Walk the dog.
- Walk on the treadmill.
- Brush my teeth or use mouthwash (nothing tastes good after this).
- Ride my bicycle.

It's a double bonus when the activity you choose to get you through the emotional urge to eat is some sort of physical exercise. Not only are you avoiding the excess calories but you are burning more than you would normally burn. Finding a solution to a problem that provides a double benefit became a little game I played with myself.

Wasting Food

"Don't waste that" was often said in our house. "There's only one piece of cake left. It's not enough to save. Just eat it." Really?

We're you ever reminded about the "starving children" in the world when you were a kid? This is emotional manipulation at its best!

Let's define *wasting food*, a concept that my mother still doesn't grasp. What does *wasting food* mean to you? Does it bring back any memories or feelings? I now know that wasting food begins in the supermarket when you over-shop and continues at home when you overcook and over serve. The waste has already taken place. Whether it goes in the garbage or down my throat won't change the fact that waste has already taken place.

And how wasteful is it when you eat more than you need meal after meal, year after year, and end up overweight, with high cholesterol, high blood pressure, and on meds? Then, I believe, what you are wasting is your good health, opportunities to do things you love, and even your life. Isn't that really wasteful?

So if the choice is to put that food in me or in the garbage pail, and I am not physically hungry, it goes in the garbage or is saved for another meal.

Period. End of story.

Bribery and Rewards

Emotional eating habits start to form when food is used as a reward or a bribe with a child. How many times was I promised an ice cream cone after a doctor visit? There would be two scoops if shots had been involved.

The only time I didn't get ice cream after a doctor appointment was when we visited the diet pill doctor. I remember when my ever-dieting aunt had a stroke of brilliance and put me and my cousin on an ice cream diet. I kid you not. She had what she believed was magical weight loss ice cream that she served us for breakfast when I slept over at their house.

It's no wonder I never knew how to recognize true physical hunger or satisfaction, or that I learned to believe that food had many different roles to play but was never about nutrition or portion sizes or only eating what my body needed.

It's Habit-Forming

Have you ever driven somewhere and not remembered the drive? How is it possible that you didn't get killed? Driving is not a natural-born instinct; it's a complex set of thoughts and actions that took you years to master. While you were learning to drive, each step in the process required you to think it through carefully, check the mirror, and buckle your seat belt. Look here, press there, and don't forget to signal. What was overwhelming at 16 years old has become instinctive by now.

Anytime we learn a new skill, it requires focus and concentration. Then, once we master the new skill, it is no longer something that warrants our full attention. Thank goodness we don't have to spend any time thinking about putting one foot in front of the other anymore. The brain files our continuously repeated, complex actions together in the back of our consciousness and calls it a habit. This is really great news when it comes to things we need to do regularly, like walking and driving.

Our eating habits began developing the day we were born, and we've been practicing what we've been taught daily ever since. Can you imagine how deeply embedded our eating habits are?

Just as we form healthy habits, we also form unhealthy habits, through practice, practice, practice. Our eating habits and beliefs are so much a part of our history that we can barely imagine there was a time when they did not exist. Can you imagine your brain as once again pure and free of any negative body image thoughts, diet myths, or emotional eating cues?

Out with the Old and in with the New

So, how do we break old habits and create new ones? It's not by willpower. That's a diet, and diets never work. We need to first become *aware* of the habit and then *change* something about the process that will cause the mind to focus on the action as if it were brand new. This will bring you into the present moment instead of allowing your old habit to take over by autopilot.

Let me give you an example. I've always been a very fast eater. I don't know when or where or why I picked up this habit, but my husband would continuously tell me that I ate too fast. Because I ate so fast, my brain didn't have time to react to the volume of food in my stomach and it never triggered the stop-eating signal until I was stuffed. I began to believe that I didn't have an off switch. It seemed like I ate to the point of stuffed at every meal.

During my weight-loss process I realized that if I slowed down my eating, I was able to enjoy the food for a longer period of time. And since that's what I was seeking – enjoyment – I could have more of it if it took longer for me to eat. I also found that by slowing down my eating, I noticed that I was satisfied with smaller portions. It may sound silly, but it worked for me.

I started experimenting with this new idea with my favorite food in the world, which is ice cream. As a kid, I always got ice cream headaches. You know the feeling when you eat ice cream too fast? Since I always got that reaction, I figured it was normal and I learned that by putting my tongue on my frozen palate it would warm it up and the brain freeze would resolve. Then, three bites later, there it was again.

But that's *just the way it was* until I sat down one day to try eating a bowl of ice cream more slowly. I started to really watch what I was eating. At that point, I allowed myself a half-cup of ice cream each night after dinner. It wasn't much compared to my previous servings of ice cream, but I was eating ice cream *and* losing two pounds a week and I felt good about that.

So, how was I going to squeeze as much pleasure as possible out of this half-cup of chocolatey, creamy goodness? I ate it really, really slowly, with a tiny spoon – the ones they give you to sample ice cream. At the ice cream parlor, I'd order my kid-size cup and ask for a tasting spoon. I would savor each tiny spoonful and my ice cream experience lasted for a much longer time than when I was shoveling it in.

Best of all: No brain freeze! WOW! I could eat ice cream and not get that horrible feeling. I still eat my ice cream with a tiny spoon.

Making this change taught me two valuable lessons: I could get more enjoyment from my food if I ate it slowly, and I would be satisfied with less of it.

Try This

If you've noticed that you're a fast eater, try eating with your opposite hand. It won't be pretty, but eventually you'll get better at it.

I used to eat with my opposite hand whenever I was eating something that I had trouble controlling my intake of, or when I was distracted by being in the company of other people. It forces you to think about each bite. Once I got good at eating with my opposite hand, I switched to eating with chopsticks. Of course, this only works if you didn't grow up using chopsticks! I would eat almost everything with chopsticks. I got really good at using chopsticks, but by then I had successfully slowed down my eating to a healthier pace for me.

In the most stressful of times, when I'm completely not paying attention, I will still inhale my food, but it happens less frequently now, I am aware of it when it's happening, and can stop it before I go too far. Also, now I know that, if necessary, I can try using chopsticks in my opposite hand.

Mindless Eating

You can eat more than you need to without knowing it, but you can also eat less without knowing it, too.

Have you ever eaten to the bottom of a bag of French fries, even though they were cold and soggy, or eaten dessert because it was included with your meal? There are many reasons why we eat food we no longer are enjoying or don't want. It doesn't matter if we're not hungry or the food is cold. We just keep eating mindlessly until it's gone, as if we have no choice in the matter and are on autopilot.

Anytime you eat, do your best to be focused only on the food and the process of eating it. When you minimize distractions, you are more easily able to call all of your senses to your food. Next time you sit down to eat, look at your food for a few seconds; smell it; notice the texture as you put a bite in your mouth. Does it crunch when you bite it? Is it sweet, salty, or maybe both?

This process of checking in with your senses is a great way to break out of your old, distracted eating pattern. Can you remember a time when your thoughts were running wild or you were so distracted by something that happened at home that you inhaled your lunch at your desk and didn't remember what you ate? That is mindless eating. Your mind was absent when you ate lunch. When that happened to me I felt cheated, because I was looking forward to the party in my mouth that the yummy burger was going to give me and yet, before I knew it, it was already gone.

There were times when I was so distracted by my work that I completely forgot that I had eaten and, since I didn't know the feeling of satisfaction from food, I'd be looking for something else to eat. I'd missed the thrill I was after and wanted a do-over. Well, I've got the pictures to show for what 20 years of mindless eating does to you.

llllllllllllllllllllllllllllll

Chapter 12
Business and Social Situations

I am fascinated by the work of Dr. Brian Wansink, whose studies have shown that the more people are at the table, and the greater variety of foods offered, the more we will eat. Psychologist, Dr. Wansink is best known for his work on food psychology and eating behavior. His work demonstrates how a store or restaurant setting tricks people into buying and eating more food than they are aware of – mindlessly, without noticing. I highly recommend his book *Mindless Eating*, wherein he describes how much more movie popcorn we eat based on the size of the bag we buy. He used refillable soup bowls to trick diners into eating more soup than they thought they had. His work clearly demonstrates how various environment cues influence

115

our food intake. The studies from his lab have been credited with the development of the 100-calorie packs.

Dr. Wansink's work helps us understand why business lunches, holidays, and vacations are challenging when it comes to eating. We are distracted by the conversation, the larger than normal portion sizes, or the social pressure to overeat and overdrink. We try to avoid these occasions out of fear of losing control, or we sometimes use them as an excuse to overindulge. Neither is helpful.

My goal is to teach you how to navigate through these occasions and feel proud of how you handled them. I don't want you to avoid going out with friends, but I do want you to be in control of your food choices and your expectations as best you can.

Meet Valerie

Valerie is an executive at a major financial institution and she travels quite a bit for work. She's on the road ten days a month and wants to lose 25 pounds. Let's look at how Valerie managed at a recent series of business meetings.

She knew it would be a long four days of meetings at a hotel out of town and she was going to be eating restaurant food at every meal with three or four potential clients. Ugh! She did a little research and found the hotel's menus online and pre-selected some dishes that would work for her for lunches and dinners. This took the pressure off of having to make those decisions while entertaining clients. She also packed a few protein bars for times when she needed a quick bite. Breakfast was simple, since the hotel offered fresh fruit, yogurt, hard-boiled eggs, and English muffins on their breakfast buffet. Having this information in advance allowed her to relax about her food choices and also be fully present for her business meeting, instead of feeling out of control or guilty for having eaten badly. All it took was a bit of pre-planning.

The practice of planning her food choices when meeting out of town was incorporated into the work Valerie did for planning those meetings. After that first one, it was part of her process for all future meetings – as important as her PowerPoint sales presentation – another to do item on her meeting checklist.

Valerie's business meeting schedule made keeping a food diary challenging while she traveled, so she did the best she could to stick with what she knew was working at home. She was also realistic in managing her expectations about the number on the scale when she returned home. Since she didn't expect to see a weight loss when she returned home, Valerie was pleasantly surprised when the scale showed she had maintained her weight after eight client meals and two cross-country plane trips. And she'd signed three new clients!

When You're a Guest

The bottom line is that you have to take responsibility for your food and cannot expect anyone else to care as much about what you're eating as you do. When you are a guest in someone's home, shift your focus to the people and activities, and make sure you don't go in hungry. Your host is not responsible for your nutrition.

Before I go to a party, I make sure to eat a protein meal right before I leave home. The protein can be egg whites, Greek yogurt, or even some steamed shrimp. My reason for this is that protein takes a long time to digest and will keep me satisfied for hours. I can be sure there will be fats and carbs available at every event, but clean, lean protein is more difficult to find. It's usually coated in batter – think fried chicken – or covered in sauce and full of fat. If I've eaten the protein of my choice before the party, I won't be tempted by those less-than-ideal choices.

Take Control

Taking along a dish that's healthy is a way to navigate barbeques and pot luck gatherings. I always take a big grain salad full of fresh veggies, a little feta cheese, and with a light vinaigrette dressing. It's a meal in a bowl, and if there's nothing else I want to eat at the party, at least I know that what I've made is healthy and satisfying, and I can eat that.

I remember the days when my ever-dieting, cranky aunt would show up with her Weight Watchers frozen meal to microwave at family dinners. We are a big, Italian family. We'd all be eating grandma's lasagna, except for my overweight aunt, who would eat a frozen packaged lasagna. God bless her, she never lost a pound, but she always had her WW frozen dinner in tow. Such a waste of time, money, and effort.

No wonder she was always cranky.

Vacation Eating

Vacation eating seems particularly challenging to some of my clients, and I'll admit it was for me, too. It's like going on vacation is a reason to overeat or overdrink, especially on a cruise where people feel like they have to eat enough to justify the price of the cruise. But who wants to associate going on a beautiful trip with coming home bloated by ten extra pounds? That doesn't sound like fun to me.

I'd rather think of it this way: I'm on vacation, so no work for me! I get to focus on taking the best possible care of myself. I can sleep a little later than I normally do. I have plenty of time to work out, have a massage, or take a yoga class, without having to rush off to work. I can choose to eat new, delicious, light healthy foods at each meal – and I can still sprinkle in a daily indulgence without losing complete control of my plan.

Plan to Indulge

I make sure to plan one indulgent food each day I'm on vacation that I savor slowly and eat only until the thrill is gone. As we've discussed, fun foods are an important part of keeping you happy and feeling indulged, but in a sensible way and this completely removes any guilt from eating your favorite foods.

Try New Things

Going on vacation is a great opportunity to try out your new habits in an unfamiliar environment. As with any habit, there are many environmental factors associated with it. When you take a new habit into a strange environment you get to see the challenge in a new light. For example, when you eat at home, you are comfortable with the surroundings and they are familiar and manageable to you, but when you're traveling you may be in a different time zone or eating ethnic foods that are unfamiliar. All of a sudden, you have to think about and focus on what to do. It can be challenging and fun, or overwhelming and scary. The choice is yours to make.

Learn and Move On

Whatever happens on vacation, learn from it. Avoid the trap of beating yourself up the day you get back home and on the scale. That will only create bad feelings, which you will want to soothe with something delicious, especially if you are in the early stages of your new habit.

IIIIIIIIIIIIIIIIIIIIIIIIIIIIIIIIIIII

Chapter 13

Lessons Learned

These Are Some of My Best Tips.

I learned a lot of lessons the hard way, and I paid for every mistake many times over. I want to help you cut through all the fog and confusion. Let me save you from making some very costly mistakes. I'll leave you with my best advice for successful weight-loss and maintenance.

Tip 1 – You Can Do This

As you begin yet another attempt to lose weight, I want you go into this process with a different mindset. I'd like you to suspend your beliefs about your dieting past and let go of all the diet myths and hype you've been tricked into believing. I'd like you to go into this process thinking that this time will be different – *This is the first time I am truly going to learn how to feed my body* – and then take responsibility for getting the job done. Tell yourself, *I am smart enough to make it through life, school, and my job, so I have all it takes to be successful at managing my weight. This is not rocket science, I can do this.*

And I believe that you can.

Tip 2 – Take Baby Steps

You've been a victim of your habits for decades and probably have gained that extra weight over a long period of time. Prepare your mindset for the fact that this is going to take time. You didn't gain the extra weight over a long weekend, so watching your carbs for a few weeks is not going to change your weight permanently. You need to approach this process with care and caution. It can't be rushed. Understand that three steps forward and two steps back is still progress.

Tip 3 – Manage Your Expectations

Managing your expectations is critical to your success. Let's face it, long-term, realistic results aren't going to be obvious in a few days. Cutting way back on your food consumption and exercising for two hours a day, six days a week, may seem like a good idea when you think it's only about calories in vs. calories out. But this tactic always fails.

You can't live that way long-term, so why try to lose weight that way?

Before you commit to any new food plan or exercise program, make sure you can see yourself living with it long-term. I'd rather you lose one pound a week and, in the process, learn about what works for you and your lifestyle, than see you drop 20 pounds in a month of starvation in a way that's not sustainable.

Break the process down into realistic goals and you'll meet them all. Bite off more than you can chew and you'll fail.

Tip 4 – Redefine Success

Is success to you a number on the scale, or is it a dress size? Be careful of how you judge yourself and your success or failure. I like to think I've had a successful day when I've been aware of my eating, journaled my food, and gotten in my treadmill time. Those are my minimums standards that I've set for myself. I don't need to be 100% in compliance 100% of the time. I'm okay with simply being honest with my answer when I ask myself, *did I do the best I could today?* If not, then I know where to focus some attention tomorrow.

Re-think the meaning of success and see if you can find satisfaction in the efforts you made rather than finding fault in the things you didn't do as well as you would have liked.

Tip 5 – Welcome Failure

So many people are afraid to fail at anything. They fear ridicule and rejection. It is horrifying for them to think they did not perform a task as well as expected. Getting all caught up in the drama of failure closes your mind to the lessons that a failure can teach you.

For example, when I go to a party hungry and someone hands me a drink and then the appetizers start arriving, it's very easy to forget all I know and just have a good old time eating, drinking, and making merry. Until the next day, when I feel bloated, my eyes are swollen, and I weigh three pounds more than the day before. *UGH! I'm a failure. Look at that number on the scale.* Then the beating starts. You know that loop that runs in your head. *Why did you do that? You know better. Now get your butt to the gym.... blah, blah, blah.* When you do this the morning after, you are only setting yourself up for future failures. You want to stop feeling badly about yourself, so you try to block out the experience and swear you'll never do it again... or you look for something to make you feel better.

Here's a new approach to try: look for the lesson in every "failure." Maybe you "failed" because you were too hungry when you went to the party. Did you save up all your calories because you knew you'd be over eating that night? That's actually how the "failure" occurred. By the time you got to the party, you were starving, so that was problem number one. Then you went in with the mindset that you were going to overeat. Problem number two. Add alcohol to the scene and now your thinking is altered, so that's problem number three. Is it any wonder you ate more than you needed?

But now it's done and you can't undo it, so let's salvage this situation by taking a lesson from it. If you can learn from this episode, then at least it served a purpose. Chances are, you will feel better about yourself if you do this, and you will probably not repeat the same mistakes, or, at least, you'll be more aware when you're in the midst of it the next time and can stop yourself in the act.

When you can learn more than one lesson per "failure," it's like finding a buy-one-get-one-free sale.

You can't depend on your hostess to be responsible for your nutrition. If they are only serving fried Twinkies at the party, it doesn't mean you have to eat them. *It's my body and I get to decide what I put into it.* For me, that means carrying a protein bar in my bag and always offering to bring a dish if the occasion warrants.

As time went by, my "failures" became less frequent. I am now surprised when I do something regrettable, but then, in an instant, I forgive myself and look for the lesson. *What can I learn from this? How can I use this "failure" to light my path?* It's all good. I'm either getting closer to my goal weight or I'm learning what not to do in the future.

There are no failures, only opportunities to learn. I find this approach much more peaceful.

Tip 6 – Change Your Relationship with Food

Permanent weight loss is a simple concept to understand, but a difficult one to apply to daily life. The math and science always work, but we often don't believe it because of our past failures. We have no evidence in our history that proves this works, so why believe it?

Once my clients see it work for them, they have proof that they can lose weight and they start to believe it's possible. At first, though, they imagine themselves fighting the cravings and hunger until they get to the goal, and then they can go back to their normal routine. This is a big mistake.

Changing your relationship with food is the difficult part, but it is critical for maintaining your weight-loss, and it will bring you to a peaceful place where you are the one in control of your eating. Once you realize that all of your behaviors around food come from having repeated specific actions for years and years, you realize the complexity of this relationship between you and food. Trying to change it is like trying to break up with a long-term partner: You know he isn't right for you, but you've been together for so long you can't imagine what life would be like without him or that it could actually be better.

Your relationship with food is just as complex. Would you stay in an abusive relationship with someone who promised you one thing and then did something else? Isn't that what our relationship with food is like when we overeat? "Oh, I know I shouldn't but it's so good." "It makes me feel good – that's why I do it." "What else am I going to do?" "But I don't want anything else." These are the responses my clients have offered when we talk about why they choose the foods they do. But check out how they could also come from a woman who is stuck in a bad relationship with a guy who is bringing her down.

Knowing what to do and then actually doing it are two very different things. Finding a way to apply the math and science to your life is where the magic is.

Tip 7 – Assemble Your Team

There's no way you'd tackle a huge work project without your team. You're in the leadership role here, and so you get to delegate responsibilities to your support team, based on their skills and the needs of the project. When the project is you, assembling a team of trusted advisors will accelerate your progress and keep you focused.

My team included experts who could give me the facts I required, my doctor, my acupuncturist, my food diary app, and my fitness tracker. There were others whose roles were to help keep me motivated before I found my own internal motivation: my trainer, my acupuncturist, my closest girlfriend, and my husband.

Figure out what you need, where you are lacking skills or experience, and seek it out from other sources. You don't have to do this alone when I'm happy to help you figure this out. Just drop me an email at Debbie@debbielazinsky.com

Tip 8 – Edit Toxic People from Your Life

Some people will not respond well to your new lifestyle. If your social circle includes people who primarily overeat or overdrink when they get together, you're going to feel like a fish swimming against the tide. You will be the odd person who orders their food in a particular way or refuses dessert or that second glass of wine. This may make some people uncomfortable, especially if they feel they have a weight issue and are not ready to come to terms with it. But that is not your fault or your responsibility. You can choose to limit your exposure to such people, or you can take the leadership role and suggest getting together for coffee and a bike ride every now and then instead of pizza and a movie.

Those who truly love and support you will be fine with your decisions. People with a different agenda for you than your own don't deserve a prominent place in your life.

You'll find yourself gravitating toward those who support you and slipping away from those who don't. You get to decide with whom you spend your time. Just in the same way that healthy new habits gradually crowd out your old, less productive ones, you'll find yourself wanting to spend less time with some people and gravitating toward others.

You will encounter jealousy from people who are insecure about their own body image. It's much easier to shoot you down than to admit they have an issue. Expect this and do not let it affect you. They will likely eventually realize that what you're doing is prolonging your life and allowing you to participate fully in everything life has to offer. They will eventually wake up and come to you for advice, or they will fall by the wayside and you'll remain FB friends, but that's it.

Tip 9 – Never, Ever Give Up

The bottom line is that you have to make a choice about what to eat until the day you die. So there is always another opportunity to make a better choice. It doesn't matter what you did at the last meal or last week. You can choose to have a smaller serving of the very same food you ate the day before and you're already making progress. Your success is not going to come from one grand gesture but instead from the little changes you make each day.

Tip 10 – Stay in the Moment

This is a valuable skill to develop and it is 100% better than trying to use willpower to resist food. The thought of that makes me squirm. When I am fully present, all of my senses are activated and I am alert, at my best, and able to fully enjoy whatever I am doing.

I use a few techniques to snap into the present moment and hope you try them for yourself. I like to check in with each of my senses by asking myself, *what do I smell?* and taking deep breaths, noticing what scents are in the air. Then I move along through each of my senses, asking them all to absorb and appreciate what is going on in the moment. This is magical for me when I combine it with the deep breathing exercise we discussed earlier.

Have You Considered Life after Weight-Loss?

Life surely looks different when you've lost as much as I have. Learning to navigate the world in half my previous body size was, at first, frustrating, but soon became fun for me. I felt like I had arrived from another planet. At 55-years-old I had to learn where to shop for clothes. *What is appropriate for a size six woman my age?* Since I had only shopped through catalogs or at Layne Bryant, I had no idea where to start.

And it wasn't just learning to dress that I needed to learn. I could now do things I never would have considered before – and I wanted to try it all. I had to learn how to walk in heels. I could ride a bike;

go to the beach in a two-piece bathing suit, fit in the rides at Disney World. It was a whole new world that I had only watched from a distance, and now I could jump in and experience it.

It was exhilarating. I called it being "born again."

Mirror Mirror

Things change when your body shrinks dramatically. One of the most confusing adaptations was getting used to my reflection in the mirror or seeing a photo of the new me. I was used to appearing about as wide as I was tall. I didn't used to spend much time in front of the mirror because, in my mind, if I didn't see what I looked like I didn't have to deal with it. I avoided mirrors, big windows with reflections, and, most of all, having my picture taken. When I saw a photo of myself, I'd tear it up in an effort to make my problem go away. I'd even destroy the negatives (now, with digital technology, that is no longer an option).

I had a hard time adjusting to the new, smaller reflection of myself I saw, and the first time I really noticed a dramatic difference in my shape; I thought I was seeing someone else. Realizing that it was me was startling at first. Imagine looking in the mirror and seeing someone else? Trust me, its freaky. And it demonstrates the power of the brain and how we see things through our own experiences. I couldn't wrap my brain around the fact that I could fit into one leg of my old pants. I had my husband trace the outline of my body in marker on the basement door so I could step back and see just how small my shape had become. I really had to work at owning my new shape, which came slowly and after lots of new pictures.

It's been over five years that I've maintained my weight-loss. Every once in a while, I wrap my fingers around my ankle and look at how small they really are now. Doing this is especially helpful when I feel bloated. It's as if I need proof that I didn't gain it all back overnight, or after that vacation. I'm a work in progress. Aren't we all?

Weight Loss Will Not Solve All Your Problems

Thinking that losing weight will solve all of your problems is a mistake. All of your problems are not about your weight. You may have problems that are exacerbated by your weight, but if you weren't in a trusting relationship before you lost the weight, your smaller shape isn't going to all of a sudden change that relationship. If you were prone to a particular behavior before, that's not going to go away by getting thin. That's not to say that you can't use the same habit-changing concepts in this book to work on other areas you want to change about yourself, because that is totally doable. But your problems are your problems because of how you *think*, not because of how much you weigh.

I've had clients tell me that they are afraid to lose weight because being overweight is the only life they've known. They have been overweight for so long that they don't know who they'd be if they lost it. Would they lose their friends? Would they become a skinny witch?

Absolutely not.

In your heart, you will be the same sweet, kind, loving person that you are now. You will be a more confident version of yourself – more willing to risk rejection, better able to bounce back from missteps. By the same token, if you are an unhappy, negative, attention-seeking drama queen, guess what? You will be that same nasty person in a smaller body.

Time Flies When You're Having Fun

When your new, healthy habits take hold and you're running on autopilot toward your goal, it's magical. You stop worrying about every calorie and squat. There's a new freedom when that pre-emptive dialog stops running through your mind. All of a sudden, time begins to fly, just like before you changed your lifestyle. Remember how many New Years flew by of promising yourself that *this* would be *the* year you lost weight? And then life would distract you and it would be June before that thought came around again. Boy, does time fly when you're not paying attention.

Time is going to pass whether you do this or not. So why not?

||||||||||||||||||||||||||||||||||

Chapter 14

My Wish for You

My wish for you is to teach you how to live your life as if you were at your goal weight now, so that you don't wait to pursue your ideal career, you don't wait to enter into a new relationship, and you don't put off following your dreams. I want you to know that you don't have to do this alone. I did, but I wish I'd had someone like me to answer my questions and calm my fears. I wish I'd had a resource for the truth about how my body was responding and what to expect along the way. That's why I do what I do now.

Coming to terms with the fact that I was solely responsible for putting the food in my mouth was a huge turning point for me. Until then, I believed that my weight was entirely out of my control. Once I learned the math and science of how my body processed the food I ate, and that the math and science worked, whether I believed it or not, I started to think that I could do it.

When you've tried and failed at a weight-loss program, it's easy to blame yourself, but the program was designed to fail. You cannot disregard your habits and patterns and expect to change your lifestyle. It doesn't work. Diet programs are designed for the masses. You're not everybody; you are a unique individual with a specific set of valuable talents, skills, and habits. I want to teach you how to create a weight-loss plan that is uniquely yours, that works in cooperation with your habits, and that utilizes the skills you've acquired.

Gathering the facts when you start on a plan is standard operating procedure, but with all of the mixed messages released through the media how do you know who to believe? You need to know the truth about your foods and your body in order to make an informed decision. We need to be 100% honest with ourselves, but we cannot expect that same honesty from companies who market foods and quick-fix diet methods. Finding your way through the maze of confusion can seem daunting, and that is exactly why I wrote this book.

Once you know the math and science around getting the body you want, it becomes very clear what you need to do – how much to eat and exercise. You'll know how to adjust for days when you're chained to your desk or in the event of a long recovery from illness or injury. This is knowledge that no one can ever take from you.

Here's a short list of what you don't need, in my opinion: cleanses, pills, surgery, fads, gluten-free (unless you have been given a diagnosis and direction by your doctor), Paleo, Weight Watchers, Jenny Craig, Medifast, Lean Cuisine, a gym membership, juicing, kale (unless you really like it), deprivation, drama, willpower, hunger, or to be on a diet.

If only it were about food and portions, but it's not. There's also sleep, stress management, hydration, and exercise to be factored into your new routine. Each of these areas deserves consideration and inclusion in your new lifestyle. They provide the framework for living a balanced life and they make your weight-loss effort more effective and enjoyable.

I make it my priority to meet my client where ever she is on her unique path to wellness. It doesn't matter what you know or don't know about weight-loss, or how many times you've tried before. I promise you'll want to give up, many times, until you learn to be at peace with your dieting past. I've been through all the data and personal failures for you and I will meet you on your path to guide you, hold your hand, pick you up when you fall and, most of all, tell you the truth.

I believe you have what it takes to be successful at weight-loss and maintenance. I know I can fill in the missing information you need to get the job done once and for all. Just imagine what we can accomplish together!

Recommended Reading

The Practicing Mind – Thomas Sterner

Fully Engaged – Thomas Sterner

The Power of Habit: Why We Do What We Do in Life and Business – Charles Duhigg

The Compound Effect – Darren Hardy

Mindless Eating: Why We Eat More Than We Think – Brian Wansink, PhD

The Volumetrics Eating Plan – Barbara J. Rolls, Ph. D.

The Ultimate Weight Loss Solution: The 7 Keys to Weight Loss – Dr. Phil McGraw

IIIIIIIIIIIIIIIIIIIIIIIIIIIIII

References

Dr. Joseph D'Antona, DAOM
The Balance Health and Wellness Center
Long Island, New York
www.631balance.com

Dr. Alan M. Kisner, MD
Kisner Plastic Surgery
Long Island, New York
www.kisnerplasticsurgery.com

American Council on Exercise
San Diego, California
www.ACEfitness.org

III

Acknowledgements

T hank you, Dr. Joseph D'Antona, DAOM, for your extraordinary skills and for believing in me when I didn't believe in myself. You were the first healthcare professional to treat me as a whole person, with dignity and respect. It was the spark I needed to light the fire in me. You continue to push me to keep facing my fears. You will always be a treasure in my life.

Thank you, Dr. Allan Kisner, MD, for taking what was left of me and working your magic to carve away the excess skin so I could finally see the new body I had created. You are a brilliant, skilled surgeon with a heart of gold. I wish you 100 more years in practice.

Thank you, Brooke Castillo, founder of The Life Coach School. I had no idea how much I needed you and I wish I had met you before I had to figure this stuff out on my own. But, as I have learned, everything happens when it's supposed to. You validated me on many levels and help me to realize that I am enough. The impact your training has had on my life is powerful and obvious on a daily basis.

Thank you to Jay Brenner, my friend and photographer, for your patience and understanding while taking my first "after" pictures. Having my picture taken was always a frightening and anxious experience in the past. Your photo session changed that for me and the pictures you took that day are a permanent reminder of another fear I put to rest.

Similar thanks go to the incredibly talented photographer, Troy Word, and the editors, writers, and staff at *People* Magazine. Thank you for your role in the production of "Half Our Size" – it is my favorite issue every year.

Thank you, Angela Lauria, for nurturing the inner author in me who has been bursting with thoughts about this book and how much I need to tell the world that this isn't as hard as some people would like to you believe. You are exactly the resource I needed to get my message out into the world, and you are the model I want to be for my clients.

Thank you, Tom Sterner, for your brilliant book *The Practicing Mind*. I hear your stories in my head over and over, and I used my practicing mind to help me through the deadlines I faced when writing this book. You are amazing.

Thank you, Grace Kerina, for your kindness and patience throughout this process. You provided the guidance that helped me make sense of the knowledge I wanted to share with my readers. You saw inside my brain and created order from a tangled mass of thoughts and ideas.

|||||||||||||||||||||||||||||||||||||||||||||||||||

About the Author

Debbie Lazinsky is a certified Life and Weight Coach and an ACE-certified Health Coach & Personal Trainer who is dedicated to helping busy women create a realistic healthy lifestyle for themselves and their families.

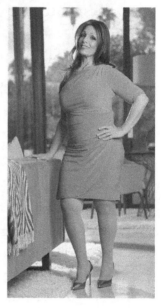

She spent 27 years rising through the corporate ranks while allowing her health to deteriorate in the process. At 320 pounds and faced with a recommendation for bariatric surgery, she decided to apply her years of corporate training and skills to her biggest challenge, her weight. Debbie was successful in losing 185 pounds without the use of drugs or surgery and has maintained the weight-loss ever since. This earned her a spot among the two percent of people who lose more than 30 pounds and keep it off.

She's been featured on numerous local and national TV shows, and in newspapers. She had the honor of being featured in the January

2014 issue of *People* magazine as someone who had lost more than half her body weight through natural means.

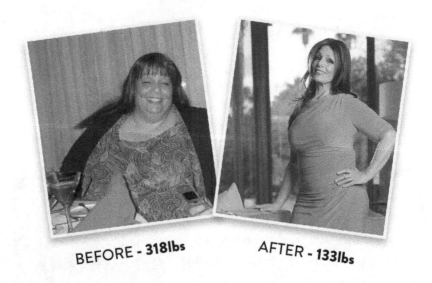

BEFORE - 318lbs   AFTER - 133lbs

Debbie teaches her method to private clients all over the world and also in small groups. She is a sought-after wellness speaker and corporate wellness advisor, as well as a passionate traveler and a great cook.

Debbie lives on Long Island in New York, with her husband of over 33 years, Neil Lazinsky. This is her first book.

www.DebbieLazinsky.com

Debbie@debbielazinsky.com

Cell (631) 813-5455

||||||||||||||||||||||||||||||||

Thank You

Thank you for taking the time to read my book. I wrote it for you because I want you to realize your dreams.

Think about how many times you've wished for a program that would get to the heart of why you overeat and can't seem to lose weight. You know that I empathize with you and was exactly where you are right now. You know you have to do something, yet everything you've tried in the past hasn't worked.

By now you may be wishing for someone to digest all of this information for you and teach you exactly what you need to know to get the job done efficiently.

I am here to help you; I've made all the mistakes for you and figured out what really works.

Knowing that my method is not for everyone, I invite my readers to schedule a free mini-session phone call with me so we can see if there is a good fit between us. I love to create a collaborative and supportive environment for my clients.

When you're ready to get to work on the most important project of your life, schedule a call with me. You can ask me anything on that call; bring me your biggest challenge.

To schedule a call, email me or go to www.debbiclazinsky.com. There's no time to lose.

debbie@debbielazinsky.com

www.debbielazinsky.com

Cell (631) 813-5455

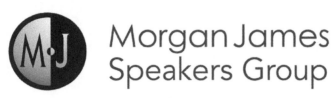

Morgan James
Speakers Group

↗ www.TheMorganJamesSpeakersGroup.com

We connect Morgan James published
authors with live and online events
and audiences whom will benefit
from their expertise.

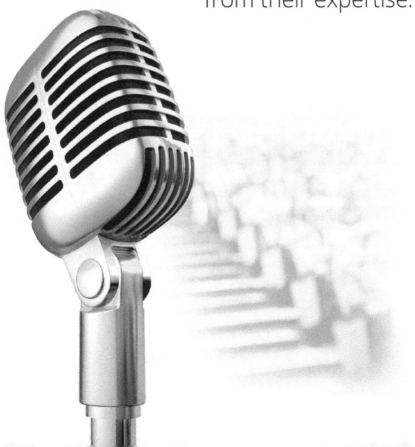

Morgan James makes all of our titles available
through the Library for All Charity Organization.

www.LibraryForAll.org

Printed in the USA
CPSIA information can be obtained
at www.ICGtesting.com
JSHW082344140824
68134JS00020B/1862

9 781683 504047